A Mental Health Workbook for Military Spouses

Evidence-Based CBT, DBT and Mindfulness
Exercises to Overcome Deployment Anxiety,
Manage PCS Moves, and Build Resilience

Katherine Sence Steele

ISBN: 978-1-7643835-4-7

First Edition: November, 2025

DISCLAIMER

This workbook is designed to provide helpful information and therapeutic exercises for military spouses seeking to improve their mental health and well-being. It is not intended to replace professional mental health treatment, medical advice, diagnosis, or therapy.

The content presented in this workbook is for educational and informational purposes only. While the exercises and strategies are based on evidence-based therapeutic approaches (Cognitive Behavioral Therapy and Dialectical Behavior Therapy), they are not a substitute for individualized professional care.

Important Considerations:

- **Seek Professional Help:** If you are experiencing severe depression, anxiety, suicidal thoughts, self-harm urges, or any mental health crisis, please contact a licensed mental health professional immediately or call the National Suicide Prevention Lifeline at 988.

- **Military Resources:** Military spouses have access to confidential mental health services through Military OneSource (1-800-342-9647), TRICARE, Military Family Life Counselors (MFLC), and installation Family Support Centers. These resources are available at no cost.

- **Individual Results May Vary:** The exercises in this workbook have helped many people, but individual experiences and outcomes will vary. Mental health recovery is a personal journey that may require professional guidance.

- **Not a Diagnosis:** This workbook does not diagnose mental health conditions. Only qualified mental health professionals can provide clinical diagnoses.

- **Consult Healthcare Providers:** Before making any changes to prescribed medications or treatment plans, consult with your healthcare provider.

- **Crisis Resources:** If you are in immediate danger or experiencing a mental health emergency, call 911, go to your nearest emergency room, or contact the Veterans Crisis Line at 988 (Press 1) or text 838255.

The author and publisher specifically disclaim any liability, loss, or risk, personal or otherwise, which is incurred as a consequence, directly or indirectly, of the use and application of any of the contents of this workbook.

Military spouses deserve comprehensive mental health support. This workbook is designed to complement—not replace—professional care and existing military family support systems.

Your well-being matters. Please reach out for help when you need it.

Table of Contents

Chapter 1: The Military Spouse Mental Health Crisis

I need to tell you something right up front. If you're reading this, chances are you're exhausted. Maybe you've been holding it together for months—or years—and you're starting to wonder if something's wrong with you. Maybe you cry in the grocery store when you see other families together. Maybe you lie awake at 2 AM, heart racing, checking your phone for messages. Maybe you've started snapping at your kids over little things, or you can't remember the last time you felt truly happy.

Here's what I want you to know: **You're not broken.**

Let me say that again because it's easy to miss when you're drowning. You are not broken. You're not weak. You're not failing at military life. What you're experiencing is a completely normal response to abnormal circumstances.

I know this because I've been where you are. Years ago, after our third PCS move in four years, I found myself sitting on the floor of an empty house, boxes stacked around me, crying so hard I couldn't catch my breath. My spouse was deployed. I had no friends in this new place. I'd just quit another job I loved because we moved again. And I thought, "What's wrong with me? Other military spouses handle this. Why can't I?"

That's when I realized something that changed everything. The problem wasn't me. The problem was that I was trying to be "resilient" without any tools to actually build resilience. I was white-knuckling my way through a lifestyle that would challenge anyone's mental health, and I was doing it alone, believing I should just be stronger.

The Numbers Tell a Story Nobody's Talking About

Let's look at what the research actually shows. More than one-third of military spouses—35.9% to be exact—meet the criteria for at least one psychiatric condition. Read that again. Over a third. That's not a few isolated cases. That's a crisis.

Military spouses experience depression at rates two to three times higher than the general population. When researchers screen broadly, 12.2% of military spouses show signs of a major depressive episode. When they narrow it down to depression that's actually interfering with daily life, it's still 6.7%. For comparison, the general population sits around 3-4%.

The anxiety numbers are even starker. About 17.4% of military spouses screen positive for generalized anxiety disorder. Some studies put it as high as 25%. And here's the kicker—in a 2024 survey, 61% of military spouses reported experiencing anxiety symptoms within the previous two weeks. Two weeks. That's not "sometimes feeling stressed." That's persistent, ongoing anxiety affecting the majority of the population.

Post-traumatic stress disorder? It shows up in 9.2% of military spouses. That's comparable to rates seen in service members themselves. In some studies, particularly those looking at spouses of veterans with PTSD, the numbers climb to 41.6% exceeding clinical cutoffs for likely PTSD.

Think about what these numbers mean. If you're struggling, you're not the exception. You're part of a massive population dealing with the same challenges, experiencing the same symptoms, and—unfortunately—suffering mostly in silence.

Why Military Spouse Mental Health Is Different

You might be thinking, "But lots of people have hard lives. What makes military life different?"

Fair question. Here's the answer: **It's the combination and the relentlessness.**

Sure, civilian spouses deal with work stress. But they don't face the possibility of their partner being killed at work. They don't have to manage months-long separations with little notice. They don't rebuild their entire lives every two to three years.

Civilian professionals face career challenges. But they're not systematically locked out of jobs because employers see "military spouse" on a resume and think "she'll just leave anyway." They don't lose $190,000 in lifetime earnings because their partner's career determines where they live.

Civilian parents struggle with childcare. But they're not doing it as temporary single parents while their partner is in a combat zone. They're not explaining to a four-year-old why daddy can't come home for Christmas. They're not watching their children's behavior deteriorate and knowing it's because of choices they didn't make.

Military life hits you with multiple major stressors simultaneously. You're dealing with:

Deployment stress—the constant fear for your spouse's safety, the role overload of managing everything alone, the emotional whiplash of reunion and reintegration. Deployments longer than eleven months create an additional 39 cases of depression per 1,000 spouses. That's 39 women who weren't depressed before who now are, just from one long deployment.

Constant relocations—every move costs an average of $5,000 out-of-pocket, takes up to twelve months to recover from financially, and requires rebuilding your entire support network from scratch. You lose your therapist. You lose your friends. You lose your sense of home. And just when you're settled? Time to move again.

Career destruction—military spouses face unemployment rates of 21-22%, which is five to seven times the national average. This isn't just about money (though that matters). It's about identity. Purpose.

The answer to "What do you do?" when someone asks. It's about watching your education and skills gather dust while you follow orders you never enlisted for.

Social isolation—65% of military spouses report moderate to high loneliness, even when they have support networks. Frequent moves mean you're always the new person. The military community can feel cliquey, with rank hierarchies creating social divisions. Civilian friends don't understand why you can't just "make plans" or why you're anxious when communication from your deployed spouse drops off for a few days.

Secondary trauma—when your spouse comes home changed by what they experienced, you absorb that trauma too. About 57% of wives of veterans with PTSD show six or more symptoms of secondary traumatic stress themselves. You become the shock absorber for their pain, and nobody's checking on how you're holding up.

All of this happens while the military culture tells you to be strong, resilient, and supportive. "Bear the rank." "Other spouses handle it." "Your service member has it harder." These messages, however well-intentioned, translate to: **Suffer in silence.**

Why "Just Be Resilient" Doesn't Work

Here's what happens when people tell military spouses to "just be resilient." You try. You try really hard. You tell yourself other people have it worse. You remind yourself you chose this life (even though you didn't choose the deployments, the moves, or the unemployment). You push down the anxiety, ignore the depression, and keep going.

Until you can't.

Resilience isn't something you conjure through willpower. It's not a personality trait some people have and others don't. Resilience is built through **specific, learnable skills** applied in the context of **adequate support and resources.**

Telling someone to "be resilient" without teaching them how is like telling someone to swim without showing them the strokes. Sure, some people figure it out through trial and error. Many others drown.

The research backs this up. Studies of military families show that resilience comes from identifiable factors: social support, household management skills, self-compassion, perceived control, family cohesion, and preparation. These are things you can develop, practice, and strengthen. But you need the tools to do it.

You're Responding Normally to Abnormal Circumstances

Let me be crystal clear about something. The anxiety you feel when your spouse is deployed to a dangerous location? That's a normal response to a genuine threat. The depression that sets in after you've moved five times in seven years and given up on having a career? That's a rational response to repeated losses. The anger you feel watching your friends advance in their careers while you're stuck in another entry-level job? That's justified frustration with an unjust situation.

Your feelings are not the problem. Your feelings are the **signal** that something in your environment needs to change.

The problem is that often, you can't change your environment. You can't stop deployments. You can't refuse PCS orders. You can't opt out of military life without asking your spouse to give up their career and identity.

So what can you change? **Your response to the circumstances.** Not because your response is wrong, but because you deserve to suffer less while living through difficult circumstances.

That's what this book is about.

What This Book Will (and Won't) Do

This is not a book that will tell you to be grateful, think positive, or appreciate what you have. You don't need another person minimizing your experience.

This is not a book that will fix your marriage, cure your spouse's PTSD, or solve the structural problems with military spouse employment. Some problems are bigger than a workbook can address.

This is not a book that will make military life easy. Nothing can do that.

What this book **will** do is teach you evidence-based mental health strategies specifically adapted for military spouse challenges. You'll learn:

- How to manage anxiety during deployments using cognitive-behavioral techniques

- How to process grief from repeated relocations without getting stuck

- How to rebuild your identity beyond career and productivity

- How to combat loneliness and build authentic connections despite constant moves

- How to protect your mental health when caring for a traumatized service member

- How to build a toolkit of coping skills that travel with you

- How to maintain wellness over the long term, through multiple challenges

Every strategy in this book is backed by research. Not military spouse-specific research (because unfortunately, very little exists), but research on trauma, anxiety, depression, resilience, and coping that has been adapted for your unique circumstances.

How to Use This Workbook

This book is structured around the major challenges military spouses face. Each chapter addresses a specific stressor—deployment, relocations, career loss, isolation, secondary trauma—and provides targeted strategies for coping.

You don't have to read this book in order. If you're currently dealing with a deployment, start with Chapter 2. If you just PCS'd and you're drowning in transition stress, jump to Chapter 3. If career loss is crushing you, go straight to Chapter 4.

Each chapter includes:

Educational content to help you understand what you're experiencing and why **Case examples** of composite characters facing similar challenges **Evidence-based strategies** you can start using immediately **Practical exercises** designed to take 10-30 minutes each

About those exercises. Please actually do them. I know it's tempting to read straight through, nodding along, thinking "that makes sense," and then closing the book. But reading about coping skills doesn't change anything. Practicing them does.

The exercises are designed for real life, which means they're short, they don't require special equipment, and they recognize you might have a toddler climbing on you or a phone call from your deployed spouse to take. Do what you can. Something is better than nothing.

A few important notes:

If you're in crisis, this book is not enough. If you're having thoughts of suicide, if you're unable to care for yourself or your children, if you're experiencing symptoms of psychosis or severe depression, you need professional help immediately. Call the **988 Suicide and Crisis Lifeline**, reach out to Military OneSource (800-342-9647), or go to your nearest emergency room. This book is a tool for building resilience, not a substitute for mental health treatment.

If you're in an abusive relationship, your safety comes first. Some of the exercises in this book assume a generally healthy relationship with your service member. If your spouse is abusive—physically, emotionally, sexually, or financially—the strategies here may not be appropriate or safe. Please reach out to the National Domestic Violence Hotline (800-799-7233) for confidential support.

Mental health conditions deserve professional treatment. This workbook can help you manage symptoms and build coping skills, but if you meet criteria for depression, anxiety disorder, PTSD, or another mental health condition, please seek professional help. Many military spouses qualify for free counseling through Military OneSource, and TRICARE covers mental health treatment.

Three Exercises to Start Your Journey

Before you move forward, I want you to do three assessments. These will help you understand where you're starting from and track your progress as you work through this book.

Exercise 1: Military Spouse Wellness Inventory

Rate yourself honestly on a scale of 1-10 in eight dimensions of wellness (1 = struggling significantly, 10 = thriving):

Physical wellness: How well are you caring for your body through sleep, nutrition, exercise, and medical care? ___

Emotional wellness: How well are you processing and expressing your emotions in healthy ways? ___

Social wellness: How connected do you feel to supportive relationships and community? ___

Intellectual wellness: How engaged are you in learning, creativity, and mental stimulation? ___

Occupational wellness: How satisfied are you with your work, purpose, or daily activities? ___

Spiritual wellness: How connected do you feel to meaning, purpose, or something larger than yourself? ___

Environmental wellness: How safe, comfortable, and supportive is your physical environment? ___

Financial wellness: How secure and stable do you feel financially? ___

Total score: ___/80

Don't judge your scores. Just notice them. This is your baseline. You'll revisit this inventory in Chapter 8 to see how far you've come.

Exercise 2: My Military Life Journey Timeline

On a piece of paper or in a journal, draw a horizontal line. Mark it with the major events of your military spouse journey: when you married, each PCS, each deployment, job losses, births, significant challenges, moments of growth.

Above the line, note positive experiences. Below the line, note difficult ones. Use different colors if that helps.

Look at your timeline. What patterns do you notice? When were your hardest periods? What helped during those times? What didn't help? Write a few sentences about what your timeline tells you.

Exercise 3: Initial Symptom Screening

Answer honestly: Over the last two weeks, how often have you been bothered by the following problems?

PHQ-9 (Depression Screening):

Rate each: 0 = Not at all, 1 = Several days, 2 = More than half the days, 3 = Nearly every day

1. Little interest or pleasure in doing things ___

2. Feeling down, depressed, or hopeless ___

3. Trouble falling/staying asleep or sleeping too much ___

4. Feeling tired or having little energy ___

5. Poor appetite or overeating ___

6. Feeling bad about yourself or that you're a failure ___

7. Trouble concentrating on things ___

8. Moving or speaking slowly, or being fidgety/restless ___

9. Thoughts that you'd be better off dead or of hurting yourself ___

Total PHQ-9 score: ___

Scoring: 0-4 minimal, 5-9 mild, 10-14 moderate, 15-19 moderately severe, 20-27 severe

GAD-7 (Anxiety Screening):

Rate each: 0 = Not at all, 1 = Several days, 2 = More than half the days, 3 = Nearly every day

1. Feeling nervous, anxious, or on edge ___

2. Not being able to stop or control worrying ___

3. Worrying too much about different things ___

4. Trouble relaxing ___

5. Being so restless that it's hard to sit still ___

6. Becoming easily annoyed or irritable ___

7. Feeling afraid as if something awful might happen ___

Total GAD-7 score: ___

Scoring: 0-4 minimal, 5-9 mild, 10-14 moderate, 15-21 severe

If you scored in the moderate to severe range on either screening, please consider reaching out for professional support. These scores suggest your symptoms are significant enough to benefit from therapy or medical intervention. That doesn't mean you're broken. It means you deserve help.

Moving Forward

You've taken the first step by opening this book. You've acknowledged that something needs to change. That takes courage, especially in a culture that prizes strength and self-sufficiency.

Here's what I want you to remember as you continue: You are not alone. You are not weak. And evidence-based strategies can help.

The challenges you face are real. The pain you feel is valid. And you deserve better than white-knuckling your way through military life, hoping you'll magically become more resilient.

In the chapters ahead, you'll learn specific, practical strategies for managing the unique stressors of military spouse life. You'll see yourself in the case examples. You'll practice skills that actually work. And you'll build a foundation of resilience that can withstand whatever comes next.

You're not broken. You're responding normally to abnormal circumstances. Now let's give you the tools to respond even better.

Chapter 2: The Deployment Cycle

Surviving Separation, Reunion, and Everything In Between

Sarah thought she was prepared for the deployment. She'd done her research, attended the family readiness meetings, and made lists of everything she needed to handle while her husband was gone. She was ready.

Except she wasn't ready for the dreams. She wasn't ready to wake up at 3 AM, heart pounding, convinced something terrible had happened. She wasn't ready for the suffocating loneliness that hit two months in, when the initial burst of "we can do this" energy wore off. She wasn't ready for how angry she'd feel when her civilian friends complained about their husbands working late.

Most of all, she wasn't ready for how hard it would be when he came home.

"Everyone talks about deployment being hard," Sarah told me later. "Nobody warned me that reunion would be harder."

If you've been through a deployment, you know exactly what Sarah means. If you're facing one, you need to know this: **Deployment is not one challenge. It's three distinct phases, each with its own mental health impacts.**

Understanding these phases—and having specific strategies for each—can mean the difference between surviving a deployment and thriving through it. Well, maybe "thriving" is a strong word. How about: between barely holding on and coping effectively?

The Three Phases Nobody Fully Prepares You For

Military families love to talk about the deployment cycle: pre-deployment, deployment, and post-deployment/reintegration. What they don't always explain is that each phase presents completely different mental health challenges requiring completely different coping strategies.

Pre-deployment (1-3 months before departure): This is when you know it's coming. The anticipation builds. Your service member starts pulling away emotionally—not because they don't love you, but because they're already preparing mentally for separation. Meanwhile, you're trying to hold your family together while planning for managing everything alone.

Research shows this is often the most stressful phase, yet it has the lowest rates of spouses seeking mental health support. Why? Because nothing has "actually happened yet." You feel like you should be able to handle the anticipatory anxiety.

Deployment (duration varies—could be months or over a year): Your service member is gone. You're managing everything: household, children, finances, car repairs, medical appointments, emotional support for kids, maintaining relationships, plus your own job if you have one. You're living with constant low-level fear punctuated by moments of acute terror when you can't reach them or when you hear news of casualties.

The statistics are stark. Deployments lasting 1-11 months create an additional 27.4 cases of depression per 1,000 military spouses. Deployments longer than eleven months? That jumps to 39.3 additional cases. Anxiety increases too—15.7 extra cases for shorter deployments, 18.7 for longer ones.

Post-deployment/Reintegration (6 months to 1 year after return): Your service member is home, and you're both trying to figure out how to be a couple and a family again. Except you've both changed. You became independent out of necessity. They experienced things they may not be able to share. You have to renegotiate every aspect of your relationship, from who handles which chores to how you parent to how you communicate about hard things.

The research here is telling: anxiety symptoms decrease after reunion, but depression doesn't significantly improve. Why? Because reunion brings its own challenges, including role conflict, loss of independence, and watching your partner struggle with reintegration.

Pre-Deployment: When the Waiting Is the Hardest Part

Jamie's husband received deployment orders six weeks before he left. For Jamie, those six weeks were torture.

"Everyone kept telling me to enjoy the time we had left," she said. "But how do you enjoy time when you're constantly thinking about the clock ticking down? Every dinner felt like it might be our last normal dinner. Every conversation felt weighted with things I should say in case I didn't get another chance."

Pre-deployment anxiety has a specific quality. It's anticipatory grief. You're mourning a loss that hasn't happened yet while trying to be present with someone who's already mentally checking out.

Your service member is often "physically present but psychologically absent" during this phase. They're preparing mentally for deployment, attending briefings, checking equipment, saying goodbye to friends. Their emotional withdrawal isn't personal, but it feels personal. You're trying to connect while they're already separating.

Meanwhile, you're drowning in preparation tasks. Legal documents. Financial arrangements. Childcare backup plans. Making sure they have everything they need. And oh yes, also trying to be supportive and keep your family functioning normally. The overwhelm is real.

Here's what helps during pre-deployment:

Acknowledge the anticipatory grief. You don't have to pretend everything's fine. It's okay to say, "I'm already sad, and you haven't even left yet." Naming the feeling often reduces its power.

Set realistic expectations for connection. Your service member is preparing to leave. That preparation requires some emotional distance. It's protective, not rejecting. You can say, "I know you need to focus on getting ready. Can we schedule specific times for us to connect? Maybe Tuesday and Thursday evenings are just ours?"

Plan for the deployment, not just the departure. Don't spend all your energy on those last few weeks. Think ahead: What will be hardest for you during deployment? How can you set up support systems now? Who can you call at 2 AM when you're panicking?

Practice the coping skills you'll need. Start using grounding techniques, cognitive restructuring, and mindfulness practices now. Build the muscle memory for these skills while you still have some bandwidth.

Challenge catastrophic thinking. Your brain will try to prepare you for the worst by imagining every terrible scenario. That's what brains do with uncertainty. But you can talk back to those thoughts.

Try this thought record:

Catastrophic thought: "Something terrible is going to happen, and he won't come back."

Evidence for: I'm scared. Deployments are dangerous. People do get hurt.

Evidence against: Statistically, most service members return safely. I've survived previous deployments. Fear isn't evidence. My brain is trying to protect me by preparing for worst-case scenarios, but this doesn't make them more likely.

More balanced thought: "Deployments involve real risk, and my fear is understandable. I can't control what happens during deployment, but I can prepare to cope with the separation and uncertainty. Most service members return safely, and I'll handle challenges as they come."

Deployment: Living in the Space Between Fear and Function

Maria's husband deployed to Afghanistan when their kids were two and four years old. For twelve months, Maria was a solo parent managing two young children, working part-time, maintaining the house, and living with constant, gnawing fear.

"The fear never went away," Maria said. "It was just always there, like background music. Most of the time I could function around it. But when he'd miss a scheduled call, or when I'd hear news of casualties in his region, the fear would become deafening."

This is the deployment reality. You're functioning at a high level out of necessity while carrying a burden of fear that never fully lifts.

The Role Overload Is Real

During deployment, you become:

- Full-time parent (if you have kids)

- Household manager

- Financial administrator

- Car maintenance coordinator

- Home repair troubleshooter

- Emotional support for children grieving absent parent

- Keeper of connections (maintaining relationships with extended family, friends, military community)

- Sometimes also employee, student, or caregiver for others

Oh, and you're doing all this while managing your own fear, loneliness, and stress.

The research is clear: difficulty managing the household during deployment predicts higher rates of anxiety and depression. This isn't about being incapable. It's about being one person trying to do the work of two.

The Communication Paradox

Here's something nobody warns you about: communication during deployment can actually increase your anxiety.

Yes, you want to talk to your service member. Yes, connection is important. But daily contact—which is now often possible via text, email, and video calls—creates a paradox.

When you talk frequently, you maintain emotional connection. That's good. But frequent communication also means:

- Increased awareness of their stress and danger

- More opportunities for miscommunication (text messages lack tone and context)

- Greater anxiety when communication is delayed or interrupted

- Difficulty creating healthy emotional distance that might protect your mental health

- Constant toggling between your separate worlds

And here's the hard part: gaps in communication generate feelings of jealousy, suspicion, and anger. When you can't reach them, your mind fills the silence with worst-case scenarios. "Are they hurt? Are they with someone else? Have they forgotten about us?"

The solution isn't to stop communicating. It's to manage your expectations and reactions to communication.

Try these strategies:

Set realistic communication agreements. Don't expect daily contact if their mission schedule makes it impossible. Agree on a general pattern: "I'll reach out when I can, likely 2-3 times per week. If you don't hear from me, assume I'm busy and safe unless you're officially notified otherwise."

Build tolerance for communication gaps. When you don't hear from them on schedule, practice this:

- Notice the anxiety ("I'm feeling scared because I haven't heard from him")

- Remind yourself of base rates ("He's missed scheduled calls before and been fine")

- Engage in distraction or soothing activities (don't sit and stare at your phone)

- Use the 5-minute rule: "I can tolerate this discomfort for five minutes. Then I'll check again."

Manage exposure to media. Limit your consumption of news about the deployment region. Yes, you want to know what's happening. But constant exposure to graphic coverage increases your baseline anxiety. Check news once daily at most.

Practice present-moment awareness. When anxiety about your service member's safety becomes overwhelming, use this grounding technique:

5-4-3-2-1 Grounding:

- Name 5 things you can see

- Name 4 things you can touch

- Name 3 things you can hear

- Name 2 things you can smell

- Name 1 thing you can taste

This interrupts the anxiety spiral and brings you back to your immediate, usually safe surroundings.

The Loneliness That Swallows Everything

The fear gets attention. The role overload is obvious. But the loneliness during deployment? That's the killer.

Three months into deployment, the initial surge of support fades. Your friends and family stop checking in as frequently. Your civilian friends can't really relate. Your military spouse friends have their own struggles. You're managing everything alone, and the isolation becomes suffocating.

Behavioral activation is your best defense against deployment loneliness and depression.

Here's how it works: Depression tells you to stay home, avoid people, and wait until you feel better. But that isolation makes depression worse. Behavioral activation flips the script—you engage in activities even when you don't feel like it, and the engagement improves your mood.

Create a Weekly Activation Plan:

Physical activity (3-4 times/week): Even 20-minute walks count. Movement improves mood.

Social connection (2-3 times/week): Coffee with a friend. Phone call with family. Spouse support group. Virtual book club. It counts even if you're not "in the mood."

Enjoyable activities (daily small ones, 1-2 bigger weekly): What did you enjoy before deployment? Reading? Gardening? Crafting? Cooking something special? Schedule it.

Accomplishment activities (2-3 times/week): Tackle a small project. Organize a closet. Learn something new. The sense of accomplishment combats the helplessness of deployment.

Track your mood before and after each activity (0-10 scale). You'll probably notice your mood improves more often than it doesn't, even when you didn't "feel like" doing the activity beforehand.

Post-Deployment: When Coming Home Is Harder Than Leaving

Mark came home from deployment, and his wife Jessica was thrilled. The homecoming was emotional and beautiful. Then reality set in.

Mark was different. More easily startled. More irritable. He'd snap at the kids over small things. He wanted to spend time alone. He questioned Jessica's decisions about the house, the finances, the children's routines—decisions she'd been making successfully for a year.

Jessica felt hurt and angry. "I kept this family running perfectly for twelve months. Now he waltzes back in and questions everything? I thought I'd feel relieved when he came home. Instead, I feel resentful."

Post-deployment reintegration lasts six months to a year, and here's what makes it so hard: **Everyone expects you to be happy, so you feel guilty about struggling.**

But reintegration is genuinely difficult. You have to renegotiate every aspect of your relationship and family life. You've both changed. You became independent, capable, and self-sufficient during deployment. Your service member experienced things that changed them. Now you have to figure out how to fit back together.

Common Reintegration Challenges:

Loss of independence: During deployment, you made all the decisions. Now you're supposed to share decision-making again, but it feels like giving up control you earned.

Parenting conflicts: You established routines with the kids. Your service member has different ideas. Who's "right"? Neither—you're just different. But it creates tension.

Service member adjustment issues: They may be dealing with PTSD symptoms, hypervigilance, irritability, sleep problems, or substance use. Their struggles become your struggles.

Unshared experiences: You each have a year's worth of experiences the other didn't witness. There's a gap between you that takes time to close.

Role renegotiation: Who does what now? Everything is up for discussion again.

Realistic expectations are crucial. Reunion doesn't mean "back to normal." There is no normal. There's only figuring out your new normal together.

Communication Skills for Reintegration:

Use "I" statements: "I feel overwhelmed when decisions I made get questioned" works better than "You're undermining everything I did."

Acknowledge both perspectives: "You experienced trauma that changed you. I became independent in ways that changed me. We're both different now."

Schedule check-ins: Set aside weekly time to discuss how reintegration is going. Not just "how was your day" but "how are we doing as a couple?"

Lower expectations: You won't immediately feel close. Intimacy rebuilds gradually. Give it time and patience.

Seek couples therapy if needed: If reintegration isn't improving after a few months, professional help is appropriate. This isn't failure—it's strategy.

Special Considerations for National Guard and Reserve Families

Everything I've described applies to active-duty families. But National Guard and Reserve families face unique additional challenges:

- They're often geographically separated from military communities and support services

- They may not have access to on-base resources

- They lose TRICARE coverage when the service member isn't activated

- Their civilian communities often don't understand military deployment

- Financial strain can be severe if military pay is less than civilian salary

- The transition into and out of "military mode" is more abrupt

Research shows Guard and Reserve spouses have particularly high rates of mental health struggles: 22% depression, 17% screening positive for PTSD, and 10% experiencing suicidal ideation 45-90 days post-deployment.

If you're a Guard or Reserve spouse, everything in this chapter applies to you, but you may need to work harder to access support. Reach out to Military OneSource—services are available to all components. Connect with other Guard/Reserve spouses online if local community isn't available. You're not less deserving of support because you're not on active duty.

When Deployment Becomes Trauma

Sometimes deployment crosses the line from "extremely stressful" to "traumatic." You need more than coping skills at that point. You need professional trauma treatment.

Signs you may need trauma-focused therapy:

- Intrusive memories or nightmares about deployment-related events

- Avoiding reminders of deployment (places, people, conversations)

- Persistent negative beliefs about yourself, others, or the world ("I can't handle anything," "No place is safe")

- Persistent fear, horror, anger, guilt, or shame

- Feeling detached from others or unable to experience positive emotions

- Hypervigilance or exaggerated startle response
- Symptoms lasting more than a month and interfering with functioning

These symptoms don't mean you're broken. They mean your nervous system needs help processing an overwhelming experience. Trauma-focused CBT, EMDR, and other evidence-based treatments can help. Please reach out to a trauma specialist if these symptoms describe your experience.

Maria's Story: Deployment Coping in Action

Remember Maria, the Army spouse with two young kids facing a twelve-month deployment? Here's how she used these strategies:

Pre-deployment: Maria identified her biggest fears and challenged them with evidence. She scheduled weekly video calls with two close friends for during deployment. She started a daily mindfulness practice—just five minutes—to build the habit.

During deployment: When anxiety about her husband's safety spiked, Maria used grounding techniques to manage acute distress. She kept a behavioral activation schedule, ensuring she left the house for social connection at least twice weekly even when she wanted to stay home. She limited news checking to once daily.

Communication: Maria and her husband agreed on a 3-times-weekly call schedule. When calls were delayed, Maria practiced tolerating the anxiety for set periods (5 minutes, then 10, then 15) rather than spiraling immediately.

Post-deployment: When her husband returned, Maria used "I" statements to express her needs during conflicts. She acknowledged her resentment about losing independence while recognizing his need to reconnect with his family. They scheduled weekly check-ins about reintegration challenges.

Was it easy? No. Did Maria struggle? Absolutely. But having specific strategies for each phase meant she didn't just survive the deployment—she maintained her mental health through it.

Your Deployment Coping Plan

Whether you're facing an upcoming deployment, currently deployed, or in reintegration, here's your planning exercise:

Where are you in the deployment cycle right now?

Pre-deployment: What are your three biggest fears? What coping skills can you practice now?

Deployment: What's your behavioral activation plan? Who's in your support network? What's your communication agreement with your service member?

Post-deployment: What's been hardest about reintegration? What do you need from your partner? When will you schedule your weekly check-ins?

Your Daily Mindfulness Practice:

Set a timer for five minutes. Find a comfortable seated position. Close your eyes or lower your gaze.

Focus on your breath. Notice the sensation of breathing—air entering and leaving your nose, chest rising and falling, belly expanding and contracting.

When your mind wanders (and it will), gently bring attention back to breath. No judgment. Just noticing and returning.

Five minutes. Every day. Build the skill of present-moment awareness that will serve you through every deployment phase.

What You Need to Remember

Deployment is not one challenge. It's three distinct phases, each requiring different coping strategies.

Your fear during deployment is not irrational. It's a normal response to real danger.

Communication with your deployed service member can both help and hurt. Manage expectations.

Loneliness during deployment requires active combat through behavioral activation.

Reintegration is often harder than deployment. Lower your expectations and give it time.

You can prepare for deployment, cope during deployment, and navigate reintegration successfully with the right tools.

You don't have to just survive it. You can actually cope well through it.

Chapter 3: PCS Moves and the Constant Goodbye

Building Resilience Through Transitions

Jennifer finished her master's degree in clinical psychology just as her Air Force spouse received orders to a new base. She couldn't transfer her clinical license to the new state quickly enough to keep her job, so she resigned. Again.

Two years later, Jennifer landed a position she loved at a university counseling center. She'd made friends. She'd found a great therapist. She'd finally joined a book club. Then: new orders.

"I cried in the grocery store when I realized I'd have to say goodbye to everyone again," Jennifer told me. "The woman next to me asked if I was okay, and I couldn't even explain. How do you tell a stranger that you're grieving friends you haven't even left yet? That you're tired of starting over? That you're starting to feel like there's no point in trying to build a life because you'll just have to dismantle it in two years?"

That's the reality of PCS (Permanent Change of Station) moves. They happen every 2-3 years on average. And every single one requires you to rebuild your entire life from scratch.

The Hidden Cost of "Just" Moving

People who haven't lived military life don't understand why PCS moves are so devastating. They think you're "just moving." But PCS moves aren't just moving.

Here's what actually happens:

Financial cost: The average PCS move costs $5,000 out of pocket, even after reimbursements. About 70% of military families pay more than $500 in moving expenses that aren't reimbursed. Financial

26

recovery takes up to twelve months or more. You're not just changing locations—you're taking a significant financial hit every few years.

Career destruction: Every move restarts your career. New license requirements. New job search. Lost seniority. Lost professional relationships. That $190,000 lifetime earnings loss for military spouses? PCS moves are a major driver.

Loss of support networks: Your friends aren't portable. Your therapist isn't portable. Your kids' pediatrician, your dentist, your favorite barista who knows your order—none of it travels with you. You lose your entire community and have to build a new one from nothing.

Disrupted mental health care: You finally found a therapist who gets it. You're on medication that's working. You have a treatment plan. Then you move, and suddenly you're starting over with waitlists, new providers who don't know your history, and gaps in care.

Children's stress: If you have kids, they're losing their friends, their school, their sense of stability. Research shows an 11% increase in children's mental and behavioral health visits when a parent is going through a PCS. You're trying to manage your own stress while helping your children process theirs.

Grief without acknowledgment: You're experiencing genuine loss—of place, community, identity, stability—but nobody frames it that way. People say "exciting new adventure!" when what you feel is devastating loss. The lack of acknowledgment for your grief makes it harder to process.

Exhaustion from repetition: It's not just one move. It's move after move after move. Each time, you tell yourself you'll bounce back faster. Sometimes you do. But the cumulative exhaustion builds. By the fifth move, you're not just tired of moving—you're bone-tired of life feeling temporary.

This isn't "just" moving. This is systematic disruption of every aspect of your life, repeated multiple times throughout your military journey.

Why Starting Over Is Actually Traumatic

Let's use the word trauma appropriately here. Not every PCS move is capital-T Trauma. But repeated relocations do create what researchers call "cumulative stress trauma"—the buildup of stress over time that overwhelms your ability to cope.

Your brain craves stability and predictability. That's not weakness—that's neurobiology. Your nervous system settles when you know what to expect: your daily routine, your physical environment, your social connections.

PCS moves obliterate predictability. Every system you've built gets dismantled. Every shortcut you've learned becomes useless. Every relationship that made you feel known and valued gets left behind.

And here's the kicker: **Just as you're settling into a new place, you start anticipating the next move.** Around 18 months in, you catch yourself thinking, "Why get too close to these people when I'll probably move again soon?" That anticipatory grief poisons your ability to fully invest in your current life.

Jennifer described it perfectly: "I found myself not unpacking certain boxes. Not pictures or decorations—those came out. But emotional investment? I kept that packed. I made friends, but I didn't let them all the way in. I liked my job, but I didn't put my full self into it. I was protecting myself from the next inevitable goodbye, but I was also making myself miserable in the present."

The Grief Inventory You Need to Do

Before we talk about strategies, you need to acknowledge what you've lost. Grief demands acknowledgment before it allows healing.

Grab a piece of paper. Write down every loss from your most recent PCS. Not just the obvious ones. Everything:

Physical losses:

- The house you loved

- Your garden
- Perfect running route
- Favorite coffee shop
- Gym where you felt comfortable
- Doctor/dentist you trusted

Relational losses:

- Close friends left behind
- Your kids' friendships
- Neighbors you relied on
- Therapist or other healthcare providers
- Mentors or professional connections
- Community groups or organizations

Identity/role losses:

- Job or volunteer position
- Expertise you'd built in your field
- Reputation in your community
- Sense of being "known"
- Confidence that came from familiarity

Intangible losses:

- Sense of home
- Feeling settled
- Predictability of daily life
- Independence (if you moved somewhere without resources)

- Hope about building a stable future

Look at your list. These losses are real. They matter. You're allowed to grieve them.

Now here's the hard question: Have you actually grieved them? Or did you immediately switch into "make the best of it" mode, pushing down the sadness to focus on unpacking and setting up the new place?

If you didn't grieve, the grief is still there. It doesn't disappear because you ignore it. It just becomes a background ache that colors everything gray.

Emotion Regulation: Processing Grief From Moves

DBT teaches specific skills for processing difficult emotions without getting overwhelmed by them or pushing them away unhealthily. These skills are perfect for PCS-related grief.

Step 1: Identify the emotion accurately

Grief from moves often masquerades as other emotions. You might feel:

- Anger ("Why do we have to do this again?")

- Anxiety ("I can't handle starting over")

- Numbness ("I don't even care anymore")

But underneath? **Grief.** Sadness about what you're losing or have lost.

Name it accurately: "I'm grieving the loss of my community in our last duty station."

Step 2: Validate the emotion

Grief about a PCS move makes perfect sense. You loved people and places, and now they're gone from your daily life. Of course you're sad. The emotion is not wrong or excessive. It's a rational response to genuine loss.

Say to yourself: "It makes complete sense that I'm grieving. I lost important relationships and a place that felt like home."

Step 3: Allow the emotion without judgment

Set a timer for 10-15 minutes. Give yourself full permission to feel the grief. Cry if you need to. Look at photos from your old duty station. Remember what you loved about it. Don't try to make it better or find silver linings. Just feel it.

When the timer goes off, engage in an activity that requires focus. You're not pushing the grief away permanently—you're building your skill of experiencing it in waves rather than being consumed by it.

Step 4: Opposite action (when appropriate)

If grief is starting to prevent you from engaging with your new location—you're avoiding meeting people, you're not unpacking, you're fantasizing constantly about your old place—grief has become stuck.

Opposite action means acting opposite to the urge the emotion is creating. Grief's urge is to isolate and reminisce. Opposite action is to engage and create new experiences.

This doesn't mean "get over it." It means "I acknowledge my grief AND I'm choosing to build a life here too."

Cognitive Restructuring: Reframing "Starting Over" Narratives

Your brain tells you stories about PCS moves. Some of those stories make transitions harder than they need to be.

Common unhelpful narratives:

"I'll never have close friends again."

- This is fortune-telling. You're predicting the future based on current feelings.

- More balanced: "Building close friendships takes time, and I'm tired of doing it repeatedly. But I've made friends before. I have the skills to do it again, even if I don't feel like it right now."

"There's no point in trying to build a life here since we'll just move again."

- This is all-or-nothing thinking combined with future-focused paralysis.

- More balanced: "We might move again in 2-3 years. But that's 2-3 years of life I could be living fully. Temporary doesn't mean worthless. I can invest in this place knowing it won't last forever."

"I can't handle another move. I'm falling apart."

- This is catastrophizing and minimizing your capabilities.

- More balanced: "This move is hard, and I'm struggling. But I've moved [number] times before and survived. I have coping skills I didn't have during earlier moves. Hard doesn't mean impossible."

"Something is wrong with me for being this upset about moving."

- This is should-ing and comparing yourself to an imaginary standard.

- More balanced: "Grief about moving is a normal human response to loss. Other people's seeming ease doesn't invalidate my struggle. I'm allowed to find this hard."

Practice catching your unhelpful narratives and talking back to them. Write them down. Examine the evidence. Create more balanced alternatives. Your thinking patterns are contributing to your distress—and you can change them.

Community Connection Strategies That Actually Work

Here's the brutal truth about PCS moves and friendships: **Building deep connections takes time, and military life doesn't give you enough time.**

Research shows it takes 40-60 hours to develop a casual friendship, 80-100 hours to become actual friends, and 200+ hours to become close friends. If you're moving every 2-3 years and juggling work, kids, and household management, where are you finding 200 hours to invest in each friendship?

You're not. So you need strategies for both building connections more efficiently AND maintaining relationships across distance.

Speed-Building Meaningful Relationships:

Join groups with built-in regular contact. Book clubs, running groups, volunteer organizations, or faith communities create structured time together. You're not starting from zero each interaction.

Be vulnerably authentic early. Skip the small talk when possible. When someone asks "How are you?" occasionally say something real: "Honestly, I'm struggling with this move." Vulnerability accelerates intimacy.

Initiate actively. New-to-area etiquette says you have to wait for invitations. Ignore that. Invite people for coffee. Suggest playdates. Host a game night. Be the person who reaches out.

Accept "good enough" friendships. Not every friendship needs to be your soulmate connection. Friendly acquaintances who text occasionally and meet up sometimes are valuable too. Don't let perfect be the enemy of good.

Identifying Portable vs. Place-Based Support:

Not all your relationships and support sources have to be local. Map out your support system:

Portable support (travels with you):

- Long-distance friends and family (phone, video chat, texting)
- Online communities
- Virtual therapy
- Faith community connections you maintain remotely
- Military spouse networks
- Your partner (when available and healthy)

Place-based support (must rebuild each move):

- Local friends for coffee, playdates, emergencies
- In-person therapist
- Professional networks
- Children's friends' parents
- Neighbors
- Local organizations

Build both types intentionally. Portable support provides continuity. Place-based support provides practical help and regular contact.

Self-Compassion: Being Kind to Yourself During Transitions

Remember Jennifer, the clinical psychologist? Here's what she told herself during her fourth PCS move: "I should be better at this by now. I'm a mental health professional. I know the strategies. Why am I still falling apart?"

That's the opposite of self-compassion.

Self-compassion has three components, and they're all critical during PCS transitions:

Self-kindness vs. self-judgment: Instead of: "I'm a mess. I should be handling this better." Try: "Moving is hard for humans. I'm being really hard on myself when what I need is gentleness. How would I treat a friend going through this?"

Common humanity vs. isolation: Instead of: "Everyone else seems fine. What's wrong with me?" Try: "Sixty-five percent of military spouses report high loneliness. Most people struggle with moves but don't show it publicly. I'm not uniquely broken—I'm having a universal human response to loss."

Mindfulness vs. over-identification: Instead of: Getting lost in the grief spiral, believing this sadness is all you are Try: "I'm noticing I'm having thoughts about how hard this move is. I'm noticing grief in my chest. These are experiences I'm having, not the totality of who I am."

Practice: Self-Compassion Break

When you're struggling with move-related distress, put your hand on your heart (really, the physical touch helps) and say:

"This is a moment of suffering. Moving is hard. Many military spouses feel this way—I'm not alone. May I be kind to myself in this moment. May I give myself the compassion I need."

It might feel awkward at first. Do it anyway. Self-compassion is a skill that builds with practice.

Behavioral Activation: Fighting Isolation in New Locations

When you first arrive at a new duty station, the isolation can be paralyzing. You don't know anyone. You don't know where anything is. Your go-to coping strategies (coffee with a friend, your favorite hiking trail, your regular yoga class) don't exist here.

Depression says: "Stay home. Don't bother. What's the point?"

Behavioral activation says: "Act opposite to that urge. Engage even when you don't feel like it."

Your First 90 Days Action Plan:

Week 1-2: Survival and setup

- Unpack essentials

- Learn basic geography (grocery store, gas station, pharmacy)

- One small act of self-care daily (even if it's just 10-minute walk)

Week 3-4: Initial exploration

- Identify 3 potential social opportunities (church, gym, community group, spouse network)

- Attend one introduction event for each (doesn't mean you're committing, just exploring)

- Reach out to one person from each event after attending

Week 5-8: Building momentum

- Choose 1-2 activities to continue regularly

- Invite someone for coffee/playdate

- Explore local area (find a coffee shop you like, a park, a running route)

- Join one online community for continuity

Week 9-12: Establishing routine

- Have regular schedule with at least 2 social activities per week

- Identify 2-3 people you could reach out to if you needed support

- Create weekly self-care plan

- Begin therapy search if needed

Track your mood before and after social activities. You'll probably notice improvement after engagement, even when you didn't feel like going beforehand. Let that data override depression's lies about isolation being better.

Teaching Your Brain to Feel Safe in New Places

Your nervous system doesn't like PCS moves. After multiple relocations, your brain may start treating every new location with heightened vigilance: "We don't know this place. Nowhere is safe. We could be uprooted again at any moment."

This manifests as:

- Difficulty sleeping in new house

- Increased anxiety or irritability

- Feeling unsettled even after months

- Inability to relax or feel at home

You can help your nervous system settle using these strategies:

Create consistent rituals: Even when everything else changes, some things can stay the same. Morning coffee routine. Evening walk. Friday movie night. Kids' bedtime routine. Consistency signals safety to your brain.

Unpack comfort items first: Don't save your favorite things for last. Put up family photos immediately. Unpack your favorite blanket. Use your special coffee mug. These familiar items help your brain recognize this as "home."

Establish physical territory: Designate a space that's entirely yours. A reading chair. A corner of the bedroom. A home office. Personalize it immediately. This gives you a secure base.

Build new positive associations: Don't just exist in your new location—create good memories. Find a restaurant you love. Discover a beautiful spot for sunset watching. Create birthday traditions at the new place. You're teaching your brain this location can hold joy.

Practice grounding regularly: Daily grounding exercises help your nervous system recognize you're safe right now. Try: feet on floor, notice the sensation. Hands on legs, feel the pressure. Look around the room, name colors you see. "Right now, in this moment, I'm safe."

Jennifer's Transition Toolkit

Remember Jennifer? Here's what her portable transition toolkit included:

Digital resources:

- Online therapy she could maintain across moves
- Virtual book club with military spouse friends from previous duty stations
- Podcast queue for familiar voices during unpacking
- Photos of people and places from previous duty stations

Physical comfort items:

- Favorite coffee mug (unpacked first every move)
- Soft blanket for reading chair
- Family photo collage (up on wall within 48 hours)
- Essential oil diffuser with consistent scent

Mental strategies:

- Self-compassion phrases written in journal
- List of cognitive distortions she tended toward
- Behavioral activation schedule template
- Contact list of portable support people

Practical systems:

- New duty station checklist (license transfer, medical, schools, etc.)
- Template for introducing herself to potential friends
- List of types of organizations to seek out (book clubs, volunteer groups, professional networks)

Emergency resources:

- Military OneSource number
- Crisis hotline numbers
- Portable therapy worksheets for hard days
- Permission letter to herself: "You don't have to be okay right away. Give yourself 6 months to settle."

Creating a transition toolkit before you need it means you have resources ready when you're in the chaos of a move.

Building Your Portable Coping Skills

The most important thing about PCS moves is this: **Your external environment constantly changes, but your internal toolkit travels with you.**

You can't take your therapist to the next duty station. But you can take the skills she taught you.

You can't pack your book club friends in a moving box. But you can maintain those relationships virtually and build skills for making new friends.

You can't transport your sense of home. But you can learn how to create home anywhere.

This is what building resilience through transitions means. Not that moves don't hurt. Not that you don't grieve. But that you have tools to cope with moves, process grief, rebuild community, and create stability within instability.

Those skills are yours forever. They're the most portable things you own.

Honoring Your Losses While Building Resilience

Here's what I want you to remember about PCS moves: **You can honor your grief AND move forward. These aren't mutually exclusive.**

You're allowed to be sad about leaving while also being willing to engage with your new location.

You can miss your old friends while making new ones.

You can wish you didn't have to move while also making the best of where you are.

Both/and thinking is the key. Not "I should be over this by now." Not "I need to focus only on the positive." But "This is genuinely hard, and I'm coping with it."

PCS moves will probably always be difficult. But difficult doesn't mean devastating. With the right tools, you can process grief, rebuild community, maintain continuity, and create home wherever you land.

You've survived every PCS move before this one. You have more skills than you realize. And the coping strategies you're building now will serve you through every future transition.

You can be rooted even while mobile. That's not a contradiction—it's a skill.

Chapter 4: Reclaiming Your Identity

When Career Loss Becomes Mental Health Crisis

David sat across from me in my office, his resume in his hands. Master's degree in engineering from a top university. Six years of experience in aerospace. Excellent performance reviews. Three p rofessional certifications.

And currently? Working part-time at Home Depot.

"I'm not ungrateful," he said quickly. "The job's fine. It pays some bills. But I spent years becoming an engineer. I loved what I did. And now I'm explaining to customers which drill bits to buy."

His voice cracked. "My wife's career is thriving. She's doing important work in the Navy. And I'm... I don't even know what I am anymore. When people ask what I do, I don't know how to answer. 'I'm a military spouse' sounds like an excuse. 'I'm an engineer' feels like a lie since I haven't practiced in three years. 'I work at Home Depot' makes me want to disappear."

That's when the tears came. Not because there's anything wrong with working retail. But because David's identity had been stripped away, piece by piece, through relocations that made his career impossible to maintain.

This is the conversation nobody wants to have about military spouse unemployment. It's not just about money. It's about who you are when your career—the thing you spent years building, the thing that gave you purpose and identity—disappears.

The Numbers That Tell a Devastating Story

Let's start with the statistics, because they're worse than most people realize.

Military spouses face unemployment rates of 21-22%. That's not a typo. About one in five military spouses who want to work can't find employment. For context, the national unemployment rate hovers around 3-4%. Military spouses are unemployed at **five to seven times the rate** of the general population.

And it's been this way for nearly a decade. The unemployment rate hasn't budged significantly in years, despite awareness campaigns, despite hiring initiatives, despite everyone acknowledging there's a problem.

When military spouses do find work, 31-51% are underemployed—working in positions below their education and skill level or working part-time when they want full-time hours. Remember David? Master's degree in engineering, working part-time retail? That's underemployment.

The financial impact is staggering. Military spouses earn about **$12,000 less per year** than their civilian counterparts with similar education. Over a 20-year military career, that's a cumulative loss of **$190,000** in earnings. Nearly two hundred thousand dollars that could have gone toward your children's education, retirement savings, or simply financial security.

Here's the education paradox that makes this even more maddening: **37% of military spouses have bachelor's degrees** (compared to 24% of Americans). **38% have postgraduate degrees** (compared to 14% of Americans). Military spouses are significantly more educated than the general population.

Yet they can't find work.

It's not that military spouses lack education, skills, or work ethic. The system is rigged against them.

Why This Isn't "Just" About Money

When I mention military spouse unemployment, people often respond, "Well, military pay is decent. Can't families live on one income?"

Maybe. Some can. But that question misses the entire point.

42

Your career is not just your paycheck. Your career is your identity.

Think about it. When someone asks "What do you do?" they're really asking "Who are you?" Your answer to that question shapes how others see you and how you see yourself.

Your career provides:

- **Identity and purpose**: "I'm a teacher. I help kids learn."

- **Intellectual stimulation**: Using your brain in ways that challenge and engage you

- **Social connection**: Work relationships and professional community

- **Autonomy**: Making decisions and having control over part of your life

- **Achievement**: Setting goals and accomplishing things

- **Structure**: Daily routine and sense of productivity

- **Self-esteem**: Feeling competent and valuable

When military life strips away your career, it's not just taking your income. It's taking your answer to "Who am I?" It's taking your sense of purpose, your intellectual engagement, your professional community, your autonomy over your own life.

And then, because military culture emphasizes service and sacrifice, you're supposed to be fine with it. You're supposed to say, "It's worth it for my spouse's career." And maybe it is worth it—but that doesn't mean it doesn't hurt like hell.

The Education Paradox: Highly Educated and Highly Unemployed

Sarah had a Ph.D. in biology. She'd published research. She'd taught at the university level. She was qualified for prestigious positions in academia or industry.

After her third PCS move, she applied for 47 jobs. She got 2 interviews. Zero offers.

"I started removing things from my resume," Sarah told me. "I took off my Ph.D. because I thought maybe I seemed overqualified. I removed publications because maybe employers thought I'd leave for a better position. I even considered using a different last name so they wouldn't immediately identify me as a military spouse."

This is what the education paradox looks like in real life. You invest years in education—taking on student debt, sacrificing time with family, pushing yourself through difficult programs. You earn credentials that should make you highly employable.

Then you discover your education actually hurts your job prospects.

Employers see "military spouse" and think:

- "She'll just move in a year or two"

- "Why train her when she'll leave?"

- "Her resume has gaps—what's wrong with her?"

- "She's overqualified and will leave for something better"

Meanwhile, professional licenses don't transfer across state lines smoothly. Teachers, counselors, nurses, lawyers, social workers, occupational therapists—all licensed professions that require state-specific credentials. Every PCS means months of paperwork, fees, additional requirements, and often a gap in employment while you navigate the bureaucracy.

So you have the education. You have the skills. You have the motivation. But the barriers are so high that eventually, you stop trying.

Unpacking the Shame

Here's what nobody talks about: **The shame that comes with unemployment or underemployment is crushing.**

When you're at a spouse event and someone asks what you do, the shame radiates through your body. You mumble something about "looking for work" or "staying home with the kids" (even if your kids are in school full-time). You watch other spouses describe their careers and feel like you're failing at adult life.

When you're at your 15-year college reunion and your classmates are discussing their career achievements, you have nothing to contribute. You make vague references to "supporting my spouse's military service" and change the subject quickly.

When your own parents ask when you're going to use your expensive degree, you don't know what to say. When your civilian friends advance in their careers while you're starting over at entry-level for the third time, the comparison is painful.

The shame gets internalized. You start believing:

- "I'm wasting my education"
- "I'm not contributing"
- "I'm less than other people who have careers"
- "I'm financially dependent and that makes me worthless"
- "My spouse must be disappointed in me"
- "I'm setting a bad example for my children"

Let me be extremely clear: **These beliefs are lies.**

Your worth is not your productivity. Your value as a human being is not tied to your employment status. The military spouse unemployment crisis is a structural problem, not a personal failing.

But knowing that intellectually doesn't stop the shame from eating at you.

The Financial Stress and Mental Health Connection

Let's talk about what financial insecurity actually does to your mental health, because it's not subtle.

Research consistently shows that financial stress is one of the strongest predictors of depression and anxiety. When you can't pay bills, when you have no emergency savings, when every unexpected expense creates a crisis—your nervous system stays in fight-or-flight mode.

For military families, the statistics are sobering:

- 40% of military families report not feeling financially comfortable

- Only 60% feel financially comfortable (down 10% from previous years)

- 52% have had trouble saving money over the past two years

- 22% have less than $500 in savings

- 35% have less than three months of emergency savings

Housing costs have exploded. Only 26% of military families report that BAH (Basic Allowance for Housing) covers their housing costs, down from 42% in 2020. That means 73% are paying out-of-pocket for housing, with many paying $200+ per month beyond what BAH covers.

And here's the kicker: **77% of military spouses say two incomes are vital to their family's financial well-being.** That number was 63% in 2019. Two-income necessity has jumped 14 percentage points in just a few years.

But remember that 21-22% unemployment rate? And the 31-51% underemployment rate? Military families increasingly need two incomes to survive, but the military spouse can't reliably contribute that second income.

This creates a specific type of stress: **helpless stress.** You need to work. You want to work. But structural barriers prevent you from working. You can't fix the problem through effort or willpower. You're trapped.

Helpless stress is particularly damaging to mental health. It creates feelings of:

- Anxiety about finances
- Depression about loss of control
- Anger about unfairness
- Shame about "not contributing"
- Resentment toward the military lifestyle
- Guilt about resenting something your spouse chose
- Fear about long-term financial security

If you're experiencing depression or anxiety related to career loss and financial stress, you're not overreacting. You're having a normal response to a genuinely difficult situation.

The "Trailing Spouse" Identity Crisis

Jessica used to introduce herself by her career: "I'm a social worker." After her third PCS move and her third job loss, she started saying, "I'm a military spouse."

"That became my entire identity," she said. "Not what I do or what I'm good at. Just who I'm married to. My whole life revolves around my husband's career. Where we live, when we move, whether I can work—none of it is up to me. I feel like I've disappeared."

This is the trailing spouse identity crisis. Your entire life is determined by someone else's career decisions. You follow where they're stationed. You leave jobs when they get new orders. You can't plan your own career trajectory because you don't control where you'll be living.

The loss of autonomy is profound. Adults typically have significant control over major life decisions: where to live, what work to do, which community to join. Military spouses have minimal control over these fundamental choices.

And here's what makes it harder: Your service member didn't choose this for you. They chose military service for themselves. You chose to support them, but you didn't necessarily choose to sacrifice your entire career. The distinction matters.

Some spouses feel resentful, then feel guilty about the resentment. "He's serving his country. How can I be mad about that?" But you're not mad that he's serving. You're mad that military spouse unemployment is accepted as inevitable rather than treated as the crisis it is.

Finding Purpose Beyond Employment

Okay, so the structural barriers to employment are real and significant. You might not be able to solve them individually. Does that mean you're stuck feeling purposeless and depressed?

No. But it does mean you need to expand your definition of purpose beyond "job I get paid for."

This isn't toxic positivity. I'm not saying "Just be grateful!" or "Find joy in being unemployed!" I'm saying: **If external circumstances prevent you from finding purpose through employment, you need other sources of meaning.**

Purpose can come from:

Values-aligned activities: What matters to you? If education matters, could you tutor or mentor? If creativity matters, could you write, paint, or make music? If helping others matters, could you volunteer? These activities won't replace a career, but they can provide meaning.

48

Skill development: Learning something new engages your brain and provides a sense of progress. Learning a language. Taking online courses. Developing a hobby into expertise. You're investing in yourself.

Advocacy work: Channels your frustration about military spouse unemployment into action. Join organizations working on license portability. Write to representatives. Share your story. Help other spouses navigate job searches.

Relationships: Investing deeply in friendships, family connections, community involvement. Relationships are a legitimate source of meaning, not just a consolation prize when you can't have a career.

Personal projects: Writing a book. Organizing a community initiative. Building something. Creating something. Completing something challenging.

Am I saying these replace a career? Absolutely not. You're allowed to want paid employment, professional identity, and financial contribution. But while you're fighting those structural battles, you don't have to let your sense of purpose shrink to nothing.

Cognitive Restructuring: Challenging Beliefs About Worth and Success

Your thoughts about career loss are probably making you more miserable than the career loss itself.

Common cognitive distortions around unemployment:

"I'm a failure because I don't have a career."

- This is labeling yourself based on circumstances largely outside your control.

- Alternative: "The military spouse unemployment rate is 21-22%. This is a structural problem, not a personal failing. I'm a capable person facing unreasonable barriers."

"My education was a waste."

- This is black-and-white thinking. Education has value beyond job placement.

- Alternative: "My education developed my thinking, expanded my worldview, and gave me skills I use in many contexts. The inability to use my degree in traditional employment doesn't erase its value."

"I'm worthless if I'm not earning money."

- This is confusing your economic productivity with your inherent worth as a human.

- Alternative: "My worth as a person is not determined by my paycheck. I contribute to my family and community in many ways. Financial contribution is one type of value, not the only type."

"Everyone must think less of me."

- This is mind-reading. You're assuming others' thoughts without evidence.

- Alternative: "Some people might judge my employment status. Others understand the challenges military spouses face. I don't actually know what people think, and their opinions don't determine my worth anyway."

"I'll never have a meaningful career."

- This is fortune-telling and all-or-nothing thinking.

- Alternative: "My career path looks different than I planned. That doesn't mean I'll never find meaningful work. Circumstances change. I can adapt."

Notice the pattern? You're not denying reality (unemployment is frustrating and unfair). But you're refusing to add self-attack to an already difficult situation.

Values Work: Who You Are Beyond What You Do

Grab a piece of paper. I want you to do an exercise that might feel uncomfortable at first.

Write your answer to this question: "Who am I when I'm not defined by my job?"

Most people struggle with this. We're so accustomed to defining ourselves by our work that removing that identity feels like removing our personality.

But you are not your job. You never were. Your job was one expression of who you are, not the totality of your being.

Values Card Sort Exercise:

Below are common values. Mark the 10 that matter most to you:

Achievement, Adventure, Authenticity, Authority, Autonomy, Belonging, Challenge, Compassion, Contribution, Courage, Creativity, Curiosity, Fairness, Family, Financial Security, Friendship, Fun, Growth, Health, Helping Others, Honesty, Humor, Independence, Influence, Inner Peace, Intimacy, Justice, Knowledge, Leadership, Learning, Love, Loyalty, Mastery, Nature, Order, Physical Fitness, Pleasure, Power, Recognition, Relationships, Religion/Spirituality, Respect, Responsibility, Risk-taking, Security, Self-discipline, Service, Simplicity, Solitude, Stability, Status, Tradition, Variety, Wealth, Wisdom

Now look at your top 10 values. How many of them require paid employment to live out? Probably very few.

If creativity matters, you can create whether you're paid or not. If contribution matters, you can contribute through volunteer work. If learning matters, you can learn independently. If relationships matter, you can invest in connections regardless of employment status.

Your values exist independent of your job. Living according to your values creates purpose. And you can do that right now, regardless of employment status.

David's Journey: From Engineering to Purpose

Remember David, the engineer working at Home Depot? Here's the rest of his story.

For months, David was deeply depressed. He stopped applying for engineering positions because the rejection was too painful. He felt ashamed at family gatherings. He snapped at his wife, resenting her successful Navy career even though he knew it wasn't her fault.

Then David did the values exercise. His top values were: creativity, contribution, problem-solving, learning, and family.

"I realized I was grieving my engineering career as if it were the only way to live my values," David said. "But engineering was just one path to those values."

David started volunteering as a mentor for high school students interested in STEM fields. He used his problem-solving skills to help a local nonprofit streamline their operations. He took online courses in woodworking and started building furniture. He coached his daughter's robotics team.

Did these activities replace his engineering career? No. David still hopes to return to engineering eventually. But in the meantime, he found ways to live according to his values that didn't depend on paid employment in his field.

"I'm still frustrated about military spouse unemployment," David said. "That hasn't changed. But I'm not depressed anymore. I know who I am beyond my job title. I'm contributing in ways that matter to me."

That's not settling. That's surviving. And sometimes surviving looks like finding purpose in unexpected places while you wait for circumstances to change.

Building Your Portable Career/Purpose Plan

Whether you're employed, underemployed, or unemployed, you need a plan that accounts for military life realities.

For those seeking employment:

Prioritize portable careers: Remote work, freelance, contract positions, entrepreneurship. Work that travels with you.

Build transferable skills: Communication, project management, digital skills. These transfer across industries and locations.

Network aggressively: Military spouse professional networks, LinkedIn, alumni connections. Many positions aren't publicly posted.

Address the military spouse reality directly: In cover letters, acknowledge you're a military spouse and frame it as an asset: "As a military spouse, I've developed exceptional adaptability, problem-solving skills, and the ability to onboard quickly in new environments."

Consider certification programs over licenses: Certifications are often portable. Licenses are state-specific nightmares.

Use spouse preference: Many government positions have military spouse preference. Use it.

For those unable to find employment:

Build skills for future employment: Online courses, certifications, skill development. You're investing in your future even if the present is frustrating.

Document your experiences: Keep a portfolio of projects, volunteer work, skills used. These count as experience even if unpaid.

Maintain professional connections: Stay active in professional associations, attend virtual conferences, engage on LinkedIn. Don't let your network disappear.

Create structure: Without employment, days can feel aimless. Build structure through routines, commitments, projects.

Protect your mental health: Depression about unemployment is common and treatable. Therapy, medication, and coping skills all help.

Financial Stress Management Worksheet

If financial stress is significant, you need specific strategies:

Step 1: Assess reality

- What's your actual financial situation? (Write numbers, not feelings)
- Monthly income: _____
- Monthly necessary expenses: _____
- Monthly discretionary spending: _____
- Emergency savings: _____
- Debt: _____

Step 2: Identify controllables vs. uncontrollables

- What can you control? (Spending on discretionary items, side income opportunities, budget adjustments)
- What can't you control? (PCS timing, military pay, spouse's employment status)

Step 3: Problem-solve controllables

- What's one spending category you could reduce?
- What's one income opportunity you could pursue (even small)?
- What's one financial goal you could set for this month?

Step 4: Manage anxiety about uncontrollables When anxiety about finances you can't control spikes:

- Acknowledge the feeling: "I'm anxious about money"

- Remind yourself what you CAN control

- Engage in an activity that requires focus (not money-related)

- Use grounding techniques

- Return to present moment: "Right now, in this moment, what do I need?"

Step 5: Seek help if needed

- Military OneSource offers financial counseling

- Navy-Marine Corps Relief Society, Army Emergency Relief, Air Force Aid Society provide emergency assistance

- Research Basic Needs Allowance eligibility

- Consumer Credit Counseling services for debt management

Redefining Success in Military Life

The hardest part of military spouse career challenges is reconciling your previous definition of success with military life realities.

Before military life, success might have meant: advancing in your career, earning a certain salary, achieving professional recognition, building expertise in your field.

In military life, those metrics often don't apply. So you have two choices: feel like a failure forever, or redefine success.

Possible new definitions of success in military life:

Adaptability: Successfully building a life at each new duty station **Resilience**: Maintaining mental health despite repeated challenges **Relationship**: Creating strong marriage/family despite stressors **Service**: Supporting your service member's career (if you choose to frame it this way) **Personal growth**: Developing skills and pursuing interests across various domains **Contribution**: Making a difference through whatever means available **Presence**: Being fully engaged with your current life rather than mourning what you can't have

None of these definitions are better or worse than career success. They're different. And if you can't have traditional career success due to circumstances outside your control, choosing to measure success by other metrics isn't settling—it's survival.

For Veteran Spouses: Identity After Military Transition

When your service member leaves the military, you lose the military spouse identity too. For some people, that's relief. For others, it's another identity loss on top of all the career losses you've already experienced.

"I was a military spouse for 18 years," one veteran spouse told me. "That became my identity. When my husband retired, I didn't know who I was anymore. I wasn't 'the military spouse' anymore, but I also wasn't a civilian spouse with a normal career history. I was just... nothing."

Transitioning out of military spouse identity can trigger grief similar to career loss. You've lost:

- Military community connection

- Shared understanding with other military spouses

- Structure and lifestyle you adapted to

- Identity framework you built over years

- Sometimes TRICARE and other benefits

But you've also gained:

- Geographic stability (maybe)

- Control over where you live

- Opportunity to rebuild a career without imminent PCS

- Freedom from deployment cycles

The transition isn't automatically positive or negative. It's another adjustment requiring grief processing and identity rebuilding.

You Are Not Your Job

Here's what I need you to hear: **Your worth is not your job. Your value is not your productivity. Your identity is not your career.**

I know the unemployment statistics. I know the financial stress. I know the shame and the frustration and the sense of wasted potential. Those feelings are all valid.

But you are not failing. The system is failing you.

While you advocate for change (and please do advocate—military spouse unemployment is a solvable problem if anyone cared to solve it), you don't have to wait to have a sense of purpose and identity.

You can grieve what you've lost while building something new. You can be angry about injustice while finding meaning in your current circumstances. You can acknowledge the structural barriers while refusing to let them define your worth.

Your career path doesn't look like you planned. That doesn't mean you've failed. That means you're building a life under extraordinary constraints—and you're doing it with creativity, resilience, and courage.

You can create meaningful purpose in this life, with or without traditional employment. Your worth has never been about your job title. It's about who you are as a human being.

And that? That's something no PCS move can take away from you.

Chapter 5: The Loneliness Epidemic

Building Connection in a Transient Life

"I have people around me," Sarah said quietly. "I'm not technically alone. I go to spouse events. I'm in a couple of Facebook groups. I talk to my mom on the phone weekly. But I'm so lonely I could scream."

Sarah is a National Guard spouse living 200 miles from the nearest military base. Her husband deploys periodically, but between deployments, they live in a rural area where Sarah doesn't know anyone with military connection. She's a stay-at-home mom with three young children. The isolation is crushing.

"My civilian friends don't understand why I'm anxious when my husband is gone for training. They don't get why I can't just 'make plans' when his schedule changes with no notice. They tell me I should be grateful he's not deployed, as if that erases everything else that's hard."

Sarah paused, tears starting. "But the military spouses I connect with online? They're hundreds of miles away. I can't text them at 2 AM when I'm having a panic attack. I can't call them to come over when I need someone to watch the kids for an hour. I have support that doesn't actually support me when I need it."

This is military spouse loneliness. You can have people and still feel profoundly alone.

The Statistics Nobody Wants to Talk About

Here's the research: **65% of military spouses report moderate to high loneliness.** Read that again. Nearly two-thirds. And this is despite many of them having support networks, social connections, and community involvement.

The loneliness epidemic affects military spouses at much higher rates than the general population. And it's not for lack of trying. Military spouses aren't sitting home avoiding people. They're actively engaged in their communities. They're in spouse groups and volunteer organizations. They're trying.

But they're still desperately lonely.

Why? Because **military spouse loneliness is structurally different from civilian loneliness.**

When a civilian feels lonely, they can:

- Invest time building deep friendships (they're not moving in two years)
- Join groups knowing they'll be there long-term
- Rely on family nearby for support
- Build a career that provides social connection
- Create a stable community over years and decades

Military spouses can't do most of that. The transience of military life means you're constantly starting over socially. Just as relationships are deepening, you move. Just as you're feeling settled in a community, your spouse gets new orders.

And that's before we even talk about the other barriers: rank hierarchy creating social divisions, fear of vulnerability when you don't fully trust people yet, geographic distance from military installations (especially for Guard/Reserve families), and the reality that civilian friends often just don't understand military life.

Why Military Spouse Loneliness Is Unique

Let me break down what makes military spouse loneliness different from regular loneliness:

The constant goodbye: You don't just lose one friend when you move. You lose your entire support network every 2-3 years. You become an expert at starting over, which sounds like a good thing until you realize it means you never stop grieving.

Rank hierarchy: Civilian friendships don't have built-in power dynamics. Military spouse friendships sometimes do. Your spouse's rank can determine which social circles you have access to, who invites you to events, and whether other spouses feel comfortable being authentic with you. It's exhausting trying to navigate friendships where rank creates invisible barriers.

The clique problem: Family Readiness Groups and spouse communities can feel cliquish. There are the spouses who've been at the duty station for years and have established friend groups. There are the spouses whose personalities naturally fit military culture. Then there's you, trying to break into established social circles while knowing you'll probably move before you fully belong.

Civilian friends don't get it: Your civilian friends love you, but they don't understand why deployment communication is complicated, why you can't make plans more than a week out, or why you're stressed about things they consider minor. The understanding gap creates distance even in longstanding friendships.

Deployment loneliness is different: When your service member is deployed, loneliness intensifies. Your partner—usually your closest support—is unavailable. You're managing everything alone. And when people ask "How are you?" they expect "Fine!" not "I'm so lonely I'm talking to myself just to hear conversation."

Guard/Reserve isolation: If you're a Guard or Reserve spouse living far from military installations, you're geographically isolated from military community. You don't have access to on-base support groups, spouse events, or the casual interactions that happen when you live near other military families. You're alone in ways active-duty spouses near bases aren't.

The "strong spouse" pressure: Military culture emphasizes resilience and self-sufficiency. Admitting loneliness feels like admitting weakness. So you suffer silently, which makes loneliness worse.

Social Support: The Most Powerful Protective Factor

Here's the thing about loneliness: it's not just uncomfortable. It's dangerous to your mental health.

Research consistently shows that **social support is the most robust moderator of military life stressors**. Translation: Social support is the number one thing that determines whether you thrive or struggle in military life.

Having people you can rely on:

- Buffers the impact of deployment stress

- Reduces depression and anxiety

- Improves your ability to cope with PCS moves

- Helps you handle the daily challenges of military life

- Protects against PTSD symptoms

- Improves your overall wellbeing

Lack of social support does the opposite. Without adequate support, you're vulnerable to every stressor military life throws at you. The deployments feel harder. The moves are more devastating. The isolation becomes overwhelming.

This isn't "it would be nice to have friends." This is "social connection is critical to your mental health survival in military life."

Quality Over Quantity in Relationships

Here's something that might surprise you: **having lots of acquaintances doesn't protect against loneliness.** You can know 50 people at spouse events and still feel profoundly alone.

What protects against loneliness is having a few **close, authentic relationships** where you feel known and valued.

Research shows different types of relationships require different time investments:

- Casual friendship: 40-60 hours

- Actual friendship: 80-100 hours

- Close friendship: 200+ hours

Look at those numbers and think about military life. If you move every 2-3 years and you're juggling work, children, household management, and possibly a deployed or frequently absent spouse, where are you finding 200 hours per friendship?

You're not. So military spouses often have lots of casual friendships—people they chat with at events, text occasionally, see at group activities—but very few close friendships where they can be fully vulnerable.

That's why you can be surrounded by people and still lonely. Surface-level connections don't meet the human need for authentic, intimate friendship.

Navigating Military Spouse Community Challenges

Let's talk honestly about Family Readiness Groups and military spouse communities, because the reality is complicated.

For some people, FRGs are lifesaving. They provide instant community, practical support during deployments, and friendships with people who understand military life. Some spouses find their closest friends through spouse organizations.

For other people, FRGs are toxic. They're cliquey. They're drama-filled. They're dominated by rank-conscious hierarchies. They feel judgmental and unwelcoming.

Both experiences are valid.

If you've tried spouse groups and hated them, you're not defective. Some spouse communities are genuinely problematic. The solution isn't to force yourself to participate in communities that make you feel worse. The solution is to find different ways to connect.

Strategies for navigating spouse communities:

Try multiple groups: One bad FRG doesn't mean all spouse organizations are bad. Try different groups at your installation or in your area.

Set boundaries: You can participate in spouse events without making them your primary social circle. Show up to the events that interest you. Skip the drama.

Seek smaller subgroups: Large group events can feel overwhelming and superficial. Look for smaller groups within the community—book clubs, running groups, coffee meetups with 3-4 people.

Be the change: If spouse groups feel cliquey, be the person who welcomes newcomers. If they feel judgmental, be the person who creates safe space for authenticity.

Find your people online: If local spouse community isn't working, online military spouse communities can provide connection. They're not a perfect substitute for in-person friendship, but they're better than isolation.

Accept it's not for you: If you've genuinely tried and spouse organizations don't work for you, that's okay. Build community through non-military channels: work, hobbies, faith communities, neighborhood connections.

Virtual Communities: Benefits and Limitations

Military spouse online communities have exploded in recent years. Facebook groups, Instagram accounts, military spouse forums—there are dozens of ways to connect virtually with other spouses.

Benefits of virtual communities:

Accessibility: Available 24/7 from anywhere. Perfect for Guard/Reserve spouses or anyone living far from installations.

Continuity: When you PCS, your virtual communities travel with you. The friendships don't end when you move.

Specificity: You can find communities for your specific situation—spouses of specific branches, spouses with specific career backgrounds, spouses of service members with PTSD, male military spouses, LGBTQ+ military spouses.

Reduced barriers: Social anxiety? Virtual communication can feel safer. Limited childcare? You can participate from home. Deployed spouse? Online communities provide connection when in-person socializing feels impossible.

Shared understanding: Everyone in military spouse virtual communities gets it. You don't have to explain why deployment communication is stressful or why PCS moves are hard.

Limitations of virtual communities:

Can't meet practical needs: Online friends can't bring you dinner when you're sick. They can't watch your kids in an emergency. They can't meet you for coffee when you need human contact.

Risk of comparison: Social media often shows curated versions of people's lives. Seeing other spouses seeming to handle everything perfectly can make you feel worse about your struggles.

Can become isolation enabler: If virtual connection replaces all in-person connection, you're still isolated. Humans need physical presence sometimes.

Drama potential: Online communities can be supportive or toxic. Some groups become drama-filled cesspools of judgment and conflict.

Doesn't address core loneliness: Virtual connection is valuable, but research shows it doesn't fully meet human need for in-person, face-to-face interaction.

The solution isn't to avoid virtual communities. It's to use them as **part** of your support system, not as a replacement for all in-person connection.

Interpersonal Effectiveness: DEAR MAN for Asking for What You Need

DBT teaches specific skills for building and maintaining relationships. One of the most useful is DEAR MAN—a technique for asking for what you need in ways that are clear and respectful.

DEAR MAN stands for:

D - Describe the situation objectively. No judgment, just facts.

E - Express your feelings using "I" statements.

A - Assert what you need clearly.

R - Reinforce why it matters or benefits the relationship.

M - Mindful - stay focused on your goal, don't get sidetracked.

A - Appear confident - even if you feel nervous, use confident body language and tone.

N - Negotiate - be willing to compromise if needed.

Example: Asking a friend for support during deployment

Describe: "My husband is deploying next month for six months. I'll be managing everything alone with two young kids."

Express: "I'm feeling anxious about the deployment and worried about handling everything solo."

Assert: "I'd really appreciate if we could set up a regular weekly coffee date during the deployment. Maybe Wednesday mornings?"

Reinforce: "It would help so much to have that consistent time with you. I know having something to look forward to will help me cope."

Mindful: (If friend brings up their busy schedule, gently redirect: "I understand you're busy. Could we find even 30 minutes weekly that works for both of us?")

Appear confident: Use steady eye contact, calm voice, clear language.

Negotiate: "If Wednesday doesn't work, I'm flexible. We could do phone calls instead of in-person if that's easier."

Notice what DEAR MAN does: It makes your needs crystal clear while being respectful of the other person. So often, we hint at what we need or expect people to figure it out. Then we feel hurt when they don't. DEAR MAN eliminates that by being direct.

The Vulnerability Challenge: Graduated Exposure to Authentic Connection

Brené Brown's research shows that vulnerability is essential to authentic connection. But vulnerability is scary, especially in military communities where you don't fully trust people yet.

The solution is graduated exposure—starting with small risks and building up to bigger vulnerability.

Vulnerability Level 1 (Low risk): Share something mildly personal. "I'm having a hard week." "This move has been tougher than expected." "I'm feeling overwhelmed today."

Vulnerability Level 2 (Medium risk): Share specific struggles. "I'm really struggling with my spouse being gone so much." "I'm feeling isolated and lonely at this duty station." "I'm worried about my career prospects."

Vulnerability Level 3 (Higher risk): Share feelings and fears. "I'm scared about the deployment." "I feel resentful about military life sometimes." "I'm struggling with my mental health."

Vulnerability Level 4 (Significant risk): Share deep struggles and ask for specific support. "I'm dealing with depression." "I'm in therapy." "I need help—can you watch my kids so I can see my counselor?"

Start at Level 1 with new relationships. If people respond with empathy and reciprocal sharing, move to Level 2. If they continue to be supportive, gradually increase vulnerability.

If someone responds judgmentally or uses your vulnerability against you, you've learned they're not safe. Stop sharing deeper things with them and invest elsewhere.

This approach protects you from oversharing too soon while still allowing authentic connection to develop.

Sarah's Strategy: Building Connection From Geographic Isolation

Remember Sarah, the Guard spouse living 200 miles from the nearest base? Here's what she did to combat isolation:

Online connections: Sarah joined three military spouse Facebook groups and one Instagram community. She engaged actively, commenting on posts and building relationships with a few specific spouses who seemed like kindred spirits.

Local connections: Even though her neighbors weren't military, Sarah started building friendships. She hosted a monthly potluck dinner for families on her street. She joined the local library's book club. She volunteered at her kids' school.

Long-distance friendships: Sarah maintained close friendships with three military spouses from previous duty stations. They video-chatted monthly and texted regularly.

Professional support: Sarah started virtual therapy with a counselor who specialized in military families. This gave her someone who understood military life and could provide consistent support.

Structured social time: Sarah scheduled specific social activities weekly: Tuesday evening book club (local), Thursday morning video coffee with military spouse friends (virtual), Saturday playdate with neighborhood families (local).

Did this eliminate Sarah's loneliness completely? No. She still experienced intense isolation sometimes, especially during her husband's training absences. But having multiple types of connection meant she wasn't dependent on any single source. When one type of support wasn't available, others were.

"I learned I needed both military spouse friends who understand this life and civilian friends who provide connection to normal life," Sarah said. "And I needed both virtual and in-person relationships. No single type of friendship met all my needs."

Mindfulness: Sitting With Loneliness Without Making It Worse

Here's a hard truth: Sometimes you're going to feel lonely, and there's nothing you can do about it in that moment.

Your spouse is deployed and you can't reach them. It's 10 PM and your friends have gone to bed. You're new to a duty station and haven't made connections yet. You're sick with young kids and nobody's available to help.

In those moments, the urge is to do something—anything—to escape the loneliness. Check social media compulsively. Text people who aren't actually close friends. Overshare with strangers. Make desperate bids for connection that you'll regret later.

Mindfulness teaches a different approach: **Sit with the loneliness without acting on destructive urges.**

Mindful approach to loneliness:

Notice the loneliness: "I'm feeling lonely right now. My chest feels tight. My thoughts are spiraling to 'nobody cares about me.'"

Acknowledge it's uncomfortable: "This feeling is really uncomfortable. I don't like it. That's okay—I'm not supposed to like loneliness."

Remind yourself it's temporary: "Feelings are not permanent. This loneliness is intense right now, but it will decrease. I've felt lonely before and it passed."

Resist destructive urges: "I want to reach out desperately to someone, anyone. But texting that acquaintance at 11 PM won't actually help. I can tolerate this feeling without acting on it."

Choose a soothing activity: Take a bath. Make tea. Watch a comforting show. Read. Journal. Do gentle stretches. These don't eliminate loneliness, but they provide comfort while you're experiencing it.

Return to the present: "Right now, in this moment, I'm safe. I'm in my home. I have what I need physically. The loneliness is a feeling, not a danger."

This doesn't make loneliness fun. But it prevents you from making it worse through desperate actions you'll regret.

Behavioral Activation: Structured Social Engagement

Depression and loneliness create a vicious cycle. You feel lonely, so you isolate. Isolation makes you more depressed. Depression makes you want to isolate more. The cycle continues until you're completely withdrawn.

Behavioral activation breaks the cycle by scheduling social engagement even when you don't feel like it.

Your Social Engagement Action Plan:

Daily: One small social interaction. Text a friend. Comment on someone's social media post meaningfully. Chat with a neighbor. Have a real conversation with the grocery store clerk. Small contact counts.

2-3 times per week: Scheduled social activity. Coffee date. Phone/video call with friend. Attend a group event (spouse group, book club, fitness class, volunteer activity). Put it on your calendar like an appointment.

Weekly: One activity that pushes you slightly outside your comfort zone. Introduce yourself to someone new. Invite someone for coffee. Attend an event where you don't know many people. Small risks build connection.

Track your experience: Before social activity, rate your mood 0-10. After, rate it again. Notice patterns. You'll probably find your mood improves more often than not, even when you didn't feel like going beforehand.

The key is **doing it whether you feel like it or not**. Feelings are not instructions. You don't have to feel motivated to engage socially. You just have to do it anyway, and often the motivation follows the action.

Balancing Military and Civilian Friendships

You need both types of friendships for different reasons:

Military spouse friendships provide:

- Shared understanding of military lifestyle
- No explanations needed about deployments, PCS moves, rank, etc.
- Empathy for military-specific struggles
- Practical support from people who've been there
- Connection to military community

Civilian friendships provide:

- Connection to non-military world
- Escape from military life stress

- Often more stable (they're not PCSing)
- Diverse perspectives
- Reminder that life exists beyond military

Neither is better. Both are valuable. The problem occurs when you only have one type.

If you only have military spouse friends, your entire social circle revolves around military life. There's no escape from military stress.

If you only have civilian friends, you're constantly explaining yourself and feeling misunderstood about core aspects of your life.

Build both intentionally. Military spouse friends for shared understanding. Civilian friends for broader perspective and often greater stability.

When to Seek Professional Help vs. Peer Support

Loneliness sometimes requires professional intervention, not just better social connections.

Seek peer support when:

- You're feeling isolated but generally functioning
- You want connection with people who understand military life
- You need practical advice about military spouse challenges
- You want to expand your social circle
- You're adjusting to a new duty station

Seek professional help when:

- Loneliness is accompanied by significant depression or anxiety
- You're having thoughts of self-harm or suicide

- Loneliness is interfering with your ability to function

- You're unable to engage socially despite trying

- You have social anxiety that prevents connection

- Loneliness is part of larger mental health issues

Professional help might mean:

- Individual therapy to address underlying depression/anxiety

- Social skills training if anxiety prevents connection

- Couples therapy if relationship issues contribute to loneliness

- Medication if mental health conditions are severe

Peer support and professional help aren't mutually exclusive. You can build friendships AND see a therapist. Both serve different purposes.

For Veteran Spouses: Losing Military Community

When your service member transitions out of the military, you lose the built-in military spouse community. This can trigger intense loneliness, especially if military spouse identity was central to how you connected with others.

"I was a Navy spouse for 16 years," one veteran spouse told me. "When my husband retired, I suddenly had no community. The spouse groups were for active-duty spouses. The veteran spouse resources were minimal. I felt like I didn't belong anywhere."

This transition requires intentional effort to build new community:

Seek veteran spouse-specific groups: Blue Star Families includes veteran spouses. Some areas have veteran spouse chapters.

Maintain military spouse friendships: Just because your spouse left the military doesn't mean you have to lose your military spouse friends. Maintain those relationships if they're meaningful.

Build civilian connections: Use the geographic stability of post-military life to invest deeply in local community. You can finally build long-term friendships without imminent PCS.

Process the identity transition: You're not a military spouse anymore. Who are you now? This identity work is part of the transition and affects how you connect with others.

You Can Build Authentic Connection

Here's what I need you to understand: **Connection is possible even in transient military life.**

Yes, frequent moves make it harder. Yes, the barriers are significant. Yes, you'll have to start over repeatedly. But authentic relationships are possible if you're willing to:

- Be vulnerable even when it's scary
- Invest in relationships knowing they might not last forever
- Build both in-person and virtual connections
- Seek multiple types of community (military and civilian)
- Ask for what you need clearly
- Engage socially even when you don't feel like it
- Give relationships time to develop
- Be the friend you want to have

Loneliness in military life is common, but it's not inevitable. With intentional strategies and persistent effort, you can build meaningful connections that sustain you through military challenges.

You don't have to do this life alone. Connection is possible. Community is possible. You just have to keep trying, even when it's hard.

Where do you belong? You belong wherever you decide to invest yourself authentically. Home isn't just a location. Home is connection with people who see you and value you.

You can create that, even in a transient life.

Chapter 6: When Your Spouse's Trauma Becomes Yours

Understanding and Healing Secondary Trauma

Lisa thought she knew what she was signing up for when she married Jake, a Marine who'd done two combat tours. She knew he had PTSD. She knew he struggled sometimes. She was prepared to be supportive.

What Lisa wasn't prepared for was how his trauma would become hers.

"I started having nightmares about things that happened to him, not to me," Lisa said. "I'd wake up at 3 AM with my heart racing, terrified, even though I was safe in our bedroom. I couldn't watch war movies anymore. Loud noises made me jump. I was exhausted all the time because I was constantly vigilant, monitoring his mood, trying to prevent outbursts, walking on eggshells."

Lisa paused, wiping tears. "The worst part was feeling guilty about my symptoms. He went through actual trauma. He served in combat. Who was I to have PTSD symptoms? I didn't earn them. But my therapist said what I was experiencing had a name: secondary traumatic stress. And it was real."

Lisa's experience is far more common than people realize. When your spouse experiences trauma, you don't just support them through it— you often develop your own trauma responses.

The Statistics on Secondary Trauma

Let's start with the numbers, because they're striking:

57% of wives of veterans with PTSD have six or more symptoms of secondary traumatic stress. More than half. This isn't a small subset—this is the majority.

When researchers look more specifically at military spouses, they find that **41.6% exceed clinical cutoffs for likely PTSD**. And **21.6% meet full diagnostic criteria for PTSD**.

But here's something important: Only 12.9% of those military spouses attributed their symptoms solely to their spouse's trauma. The rest had their own primary traumas from military life—deployments, relocations, financial stress, social isolation, loss of career and identity. So military spouses are experiencing both primary trauma from military lifestyle AND secondary trauma from their service member's experiences.

Your trauma is real. Whether it came from absorbing your spouse's experiences or from your own military life challenges, it deserves recognition and treatment.

What Is Secondary Traumatic Stress?

Secondary traumatic stress (also called vicarious trauma or compassion fatigue) occurs when you're exposed to another person's trauma and develop trauma symptoms yourself.

It's different from "being stressed about your spouse's PTSD." It's **developing actual trauma symptoms from exposure to their traumatic experiences and ongoing trauma responses.**

Common symptoms of secondary traumatic stress:

Re-experiencing symptoms:

- Nightmares about your spouse's traumatic experiences (even though you weren't there)

- Intrusive thoughts about what they went through

- Flashbacks to times when your spouse was symptomatic or in crisis

- Intense emotional distress when reminded of their trauma

Avoidance symptoms:

- Avoiding conversations about their deployment or combat experiences

- Avoiding war movies, news about military conflicts, or other trauma reminders

- Avoiding situations that might trigger your spouse (which limits your own life)

- Emotional numbing—feeling detached from your own emotions

Hyperarousal symptoms:

- Constant vigilance, monitoring your spouse's mood

- Exaggerated startle response

- Difficulty sleeping

- Irritability or angry outbursts

- Difficulty concentrating

Negative changes in mood and cognition:

- Persistent negative beliefs about yourself, others, or the world ("Nowhere is safe," "I can't trust anyone")

- Distorted blame of self or others

- Persistent negative emotional state

- Inability to experience positive emotions

- Feeling detached from others

Physical symptoms:

- Chronic fatigue

- Headaches

- Digestive issues

- Weakened immune system

- Physical tension

If you're reading this list and thinking "That's me," you're not imagining it. Secondary trauma is real, and it's common among military spouses.

How Secondary Trauma Is Different From (and Similar To) PTSD

Secondary traumatic stress and PTSD have similar symptom profiles because they're both trauma responses. The main difference is the source:

PTSD: Develops from experiencing or witnessing trauma directly

Secondary traumatic stress: Develops from exposure to someone else's trauma and their ongoing trauma symptoms

But functionally? The symptoms and their impact are similar. Your nervous system doesn't distinguish between "I experienced this" and "I'm constantly exposed to someone whose nervous system is traumatized." Either way, your own nervous system becomes dysregulated.

Here's what's important: **Secondary trauma is not less valid than primary trauma.** You don't have to have served in combat to develop trauma symptoms. Living with someone who has severe PTSD, absorbing their experiences, managing their symptoms, and living in constant state of hypervigilance—that's genuinely traumatizing.

The Caregiver Burden: When You Become the Entire Support System

Military spouses of service members with PTSD often become de facto caregivers. You're managing:

Their symptoms:

- Monitoring mood changes

- Anticipating triggers
- Managing their anger or irritability
- Dealing with nightmares, hypervigilance, avoidance
- Encouraging (or forcing) treatment engagement
- Managing medication compliance

Household responsibilities:

- Everything you already managed during deployments, except now they're home but can't fully participate
- Protecting children from spouse's symptoms
- Managing finances if their PTSD affects employment
- Maintaining household when your spouse can't contribute consistently

Your own mental health:

- Processing your own secondary trauma symptoms
- Managing anxiety about their wellbeing
- Dealing with your own triggers and hypervigilance
- Finding time for your own therapy and self-care (which often gets deprioritized)

The relationship:

- Trying to maintain intimacy when your spouse is emotionally disconnected
- Managing your own needs when your spouse can't meet them
- Feeling more like a caregiver than a partner

The caregiver burden is exhausting. And it's relentless. Unlike professional caregivers who clock out after their shift, you're on duty 24/7. There's no break from monitoring, managing, and absorbing.

Compassion Fatigue: Why You Can't Pour From an Empty Cup

Compassion fatigue is what happens when caregiving depletes you beyond your capacity to recover.

In the beginning, you have compassion and energy to support your spouse. You understand they're struggling. You want to help. You have empathy for their pain.

Over time, without adequate support and replenishment, your compassion reserves deplete. You become:

- Emotionally numb
- Resentful
- Unable to feel empathy (even though you want to)
- Detached from your spouse's struggles
- Guilty about your lack of compassion

Compassion fatigue isn't a character flaw. It's what happens when you give more than you have without replenishing yourself.

Think of it like a bank account. Caregiving is a withdrawal. Self-care, support, rest, and positive experiences are deposits. If you're constantly withdrawing without depositing, you eventually overdraft. Your compassion account hits zero.

The answer isn't "try harder to be compassionate." The answer is: **Make deposits. Replenish yourself.**

The Lost Partner: When Your Service Member Can't Support You Emotionally

This is one of the hardest parts of living with a spouse with PTSD: **The person who should be your primary emotional support is unavailable.**

In healthy relationships, both partners support each other. When you're struggling, your partner is there for you. When they're struggling, you're there for them. There's reciprocity.

When your spouse has severe PTSD, that reciprocity often disappears. They're so consumed by their own symptoms that they have nothing left to give you. They're emotionally unavailable, easily overwhelmed by others' emotions, or so detached they don't notice you're struggling.

So you're dealing with:

- Your own secondary trauma symptoms
- The stress of caregiving
- All the regular military life challenges
- WITHOUT emotional support from your primary relationship

Where does that leave you? Isolated. Exhausted. Resentful. And probably feeling guilty about the resentment.

"I know his PTSD isn't his fault," one spouse told me. "I know he didn't ask for this. But I'm drowning, and he doesn't even notice. I need support too, but there's nobody to support me. I feel completely alone."

This is a legitimate grief. You've lost the partner you thought you'd have. Yes, they're still physically present. But the emotional partnership is gone or severely limited. That loss deserves acknowledgment.

Impact on Intimacy and Relationship

PTSD affects intimacy in multiple ways:

Emotional intimacy:

- Your spouse may be emotionally numb or avoidant

- Difficulty with vulnerability and emotional connection

- Inability to engage in deep conversations

- Detachment that makes you feel alone even when together

Physical intimacy:

- Trauma can affect sexual functioning

- Hypervigilance makes physical touch uncomfortable

- Survivors of sexual trauma may struggle with any physical intimacy

- Your own trauma symptoms may affect your desire or comfort with intimacy

Trust and safety:

- If your spouse has anger issues, you may not feel safe

- Unpredictability in their mood creates walking-on-eggshells dynamic

- Difficulty trusting they won't explode or shut down

Role confusion:

- When you're functioning more as caregiver than partner, intimacy suffers

- Hard to feel romantic toward someone you're parenting or managing

- Power dynamic shifts when one person is highly symptomatic

These impacts are real. You're allowed to grieve the intimate partnership you expected to have. You're allowed to feel frustrated, sad, or resentful about these changes.

Setting Boundaries in the Caregiving Role

Here's something caregivers often resist: **You need boundaries around caregiving, even when your spouse has PTSD.**

Boundaries don't mean you don't care. Boundaries mean you're protecting your own mental health so you can continue functioning.

Examples of necessary boundaries:

"I will support you, but I won't be your only support."

- Your spouse needs professional help. You can encourage treatment and support them through it, but you can't be their therapist.

- They need their own support network (therapy, support groups, veteran peer support)

"I will help manage your symptoms, but I won't take responsibility for them."

- You can remind them to take medication, but ultimately it's their responsibility

- You can point out when their PTSD is affecting the family, but you can't control their symptoms

- Their recovery is their work, not yours

"I will accommodate some triggers, but I won't eliminate all potential triggers from our life."

- Reasonable accommodations are fine (avoiding fireworks if that's triggering)

- Unreasonable restrictions aren't sustainable (never leaving the house because crowds are triggering)

- Your life matters too

"I will be compassionate, but I won't accept abuse."

- PTSD doesn't excuse verbal, physical, or emotional abuse

- Your safety and your children's safety are non-negotiable

- Anger is a symptom; abuse is a choice

"I will support your treatment, but I have my own mental health needs."

- You deserve therapy too

- You deserve time for self-care

- Your mental health matters as much as theirs

These boundaries feel selfish when you set them. They're not. They're survival.

Lisa's Story: Healing While Still Supporting

Remember Lisa, the Marine spouse dealing with secondary trauma? Here's how she started healing:

Step 1: Acknowledging her own trauma. Lisa stopped minimizing her symptoms. She accepted that secondary traumatic stress was real and deserved treatment.

Step 2: Starting her own therapy. Lisa found a therapist who specialized in trauma and military families. For the first time, she had space to process her own experiences without prioritizing Jake's needs.

Step 3: Setting boundaries. Lisa told Jake: "I love you and I support your recovery. But I need you to take primary responsibility for managing your symptoms. I'll help, but I can't be your only support."

Step 4: Building her own support system. Lisa joined a support group for spouses of veterans with PTSD. Having others who understood made her feel less alone.

Step 5: Scheduling self-care non-negotiably. Lisa blocked out time each week for activities that replenished her: therapy, exercise, coffee with friends, reading. She stopped canceling these when Jake had a bad day.

Step 6: Trauma-focused treatment for herself. Lisa's therapist used cognitive processing therapy adapted for secondary trauma. Lisa processed her own trauma symptoms, not just her reactions to Jake's.

Step 7: Couples therapy. Once both Lisa and Jake were in individual treatment, they started couples therapy to address relationship issues caused by PTSD.

Did these steps fix everything? No. Jake still has PTSD. Lisa still has secondary trauma symptoms. But Lisa is no longer drowning. She has tools to cope, support to rely on, and boundaries that protect her mental health.

Trauma-Informed Approaches for Your Healing

If you have secondary trauma, you need trauma-focused treatment. Not just general therapy. Not just "coping with stress." Actual trauma treatment.

Effective trauma treatments include:

Cognitive Processing Therapy (CPT):

- Helps you process stuck thoughts about the trauma
- Addresses beliefs like "I should have prevented this" or "It's my fault he's struggling"
- Particularly good for guilt and self-blame

Eye Movement Desensitization and Reprocessing (EMDR):

- Processes traumatic memories through bilateral stimulation
- Effective for both primary and secondary trauma
- Reduces intensity of trauma memories and associated distress

Prolonged Exposure (PE):

- Involves gradually confronting trauma-related thoughts, feelings, and situations you've been avoiding

- Reduces avoidance and helps process trauma memories

Trauma-focused CBT:

- Combines cognitive restructuring with exposure techniques

- Addresses trauma-related thoughts and behaviors

- Teaches coping skills for managing trauma symptoms

Somatic approaches:

- Trauma is stored in the body, not just the mind

- Somatic experiencing, yoga, and body-based therapies help release stored trauma

- Particularly helpful when you have physical symptoms

Group therapy for military spouses:

- Connect with others experiencing secondary trauma

- Reduces isolation and shame

- Provides validation and practical coping strategies

You might feel guilty seeking trauma treatment when your spouse is "the one who actually served." Let go of that guilt. Your trauma is real. You deserve healing.

Cognitive Processing: Understanding Trauma Responses

Part of healing from secondary trauma involves understanding what trauma does to your nervous system and your thinking.

Common trauma-related thoughts that need processing:

"I should be able to handle this better."

- This assumes superhuman capacity. You're human. Chronic exposure to a traumatized partner affects you.

- Alternative: "I'm responding normally to abnormal circumstances. Secondary trauma is expected in my situation."

"It's selfish to focus on my needs when he's the one who served."

- This creates hierarchy of suffering where only the service member's trauma counts.

- Alternative: "We both have trauma. We both deserve healing. My mental health matters too."

"If I set boundaries, I'm abandoning him."

- This confuses boundaries with rejection.

- Alternative: "Boundaries protect my mental health so I can continue being in this relationship. I'm not abandoning him—I'm ensuring I can stay present."

"I can't trust anyone. The world isn't safe."

- This is a trauma response—hypervigilance extended to all situations.

- Alternative: "My spouse experienced trauma that makes the world feel unsafe. But I can evaluate actual risk in each situation rather than assuming everything is dangerous."

"His PTSD is my fault."

- This is irrational self-blame, common in trauma.

- Alternative: "Combat caused his PTSD. I didn't cause it, I can't control it, and I can't cure it. I can only support him while also caring for myself."

Cognitive processing involves examining these thoughts, looking at evidence, and developing more balanced perspectives.

Emotion Regulation: Managing Triggered States

When you have secondary trauma, you get triggered by things related to your spouse's trauma or their symptoms.

Maybe it's hearing fireworks (reminds you of his combat trauma). Maybe it's seeing him start to escalate (you go immediately into high alert). Maybe it's news coverage of military conflicts (triggers your fear for his wellbeing).

Emotion regulation skills for managing triggers:

Recognize the trigger: "I'm triggered right now. The fireworks are reminding me of Jake's combat trauma and his PTSD symptoms."

Name the emotion: "I'm feeling intense anxiety. My heart is racing. I want to flee or shut down."

Validate the emotion: "It makes sense I'm anxious. I've been conditioned to associate loud noises with Jake's distress. My nervous system is trying to protect me."

Use grounding: Engage your five senses to return to present moment. "Right now, I'm safe. These are fireworks, not gunfire. Jake is okay. I'm okay."

Implement coping skills:

- Paced breathing

- Progressive muscle relaxation

- Physical movement (walk, stretch)

- Cold water on face (activates parasympathetic nervous system)

- Call a support person

Opposite action (if needed): If the emotion is urging you to avoid something you actually need to do, act opposite to that urge while using coping skills.

Self-compassion: "This is hard. I'm doing the best I can. I'm healing, and healing isn't linear."

The goal isn't to never be triggered. The goal is to manage triggers when they occur without being overwhelmed by them.

Self-Compassion for Caregivers

Caregivers are often terrible at self-compassion. You judge yourself harshly for:

- Feeling resentful
- Not being endlessly patient
- Having your own needs
- Wanting breaks from caregiving
- Feeling compassion fatigue
- Sometimes wishing your life was different

All of these are normal human responses to caregiving burden. You're allowed to have them.

Self-compassion practice for caregivers:

Self-kindness: Talk to yourself the way you'd talk to a friend in your situation. Would you tell a friend she's selfish for needing breaks? No. Don't tell yourself that either.

Common humanity: Remember you're not alone in struggling with this. Caregiving for someone with PTSD is objectively difficult. Most people in your situation struggle similarly.

Mindfulness: Notice your difficult feelings without over-identifying with them. "I'm having the thought that I'm a bad spouse. That's a thought, not a fact. I'm having feelings of resentment. That's a feeling, not a character flaw."

Permission-giving: Give yourself explicit permission:

- "I'm allowed to feel frustrated"

- "I'm allowed to want time away from caregiving"

- "I'm allowed to prioritize my mental health"

- "I'm allowed to have needs, even when my spouse is struggling"

When you practice self-compassion, you're not being self-indulgent. You're being realistic about human limitations.

Couples Strategies: When and How to Address Together

Individual treatment for both partners is essential. But sometimes couples therapy is also needed to address relationship issues caused by PTSD and secondary trauma.

When to consider couples therapy:

- Communication has broken down

- Intimacy issues are significant

- You're stuck in negative patterns (criticism, defensiveness, stonewalling)

- Your spouse doesn't understand how their PTSD affects you

- You need help renegotiating roles and expectations

- Relationship distress is high on both sides

What to look for in couples therapist:

- Experience with trauma and PTSD

- Understanding of military culture

- Training in evidence-based couples therapy (Cognitive-Behavioral Conjoint Therapy, Emotionally Focused Therapy, Gottman Method)

- Ability to balance both partners' needs

- Trauma-informed approach

What couples therapy can address:

- Improving communication about PTSD symptoms and impacts
- Teaching both partners de-escalation skills
- Rebuilding intimacy and trust
- Renegotiating relationship roles
- Helping both partners understand each other's experiences
- Creating shared goals for relationship and recovery

Couples therapy isn't a substitute for individual trauma treatment. Both partners need their own therapists plus couples work.

For Veteran Spouses: Long-Term Caregiving

When your service member transitions out of the military, you might think PTSD symptoms will improve. Sometimes they do. Often they don't, or they worsen.

The structure of military life can actually help manage PTSD symptoms. Without that structure, symptoms may intensify. Additionally, transition itself is stressful, which can exacerbate PTSD.

For veteran spouses, secondary trauma becomes long-term reality. You're not just supporting them through deployment recovery. You're living with chronic PTSD, potentially for decades.

This requires different thinking:

Accept chronicity: His PTSD may never fully resolve. You're not waiting for him to "get better" before your life starts. This is your life.

Build sustainable systems: What support do you need long-term? Not just "until he recovers" but potentially indefinitely?

Protect your identity: Don't let "caregiver" become your entire identity. You're a person with needs, goals, and identity beyond supporting your spouse.

Consider VA programs: Program of Comprehensive Assistance for Family Caregivers (PCAFC) provides stipend, health insurance, respite care, and mental health counseling for eligible veteran spouse caregivers. Check eligibility.

Plan for respite: Regular breaks from caregiving are essential. Schedule them. Don't feel guilty about them.

Your Trauma Is Valid Too

Here's what I need you to hear: **Your trauma is real and valid, even if you didn't serve in combat.**

You don't need to earn trauma symptoms. You don't need to justify why secondary traumatic stress is affecting you. You don't need to minimize your experience because "others have it worse."

Living with someone with severe PTSD is traumatizing. Absorbing their trauma through proximity and caregiving is traumatizing. Military life itself—the deployments, the uncertainty, the losses—is traumatizing.

Your symptoms are not weakness. They're normal responses to abnormal stress and repeated trauma exposure.

You deserve treatment. You deserve support. You deserve healing.

And here's the paradox: **Healing yourself makes you better able to support your spouse.** When you're less depleted, less traumatized, less overwhelmed, you have more capacity for compassion. Taking care of yourself isn't selfish—it's strategic.

You can heal while still supporting your spouse. These aren't mutually exclusive. You just need to recognize that you both need healing, and you both deserve it.

Your trauma is real. Your pain is valid. And healing is possible, even while staying in the relationship.

You don't have to keep drowning to prove your love.

Chapter 7: The Practical Toolkit

Evidence-Based Skills for Daily Life

Rachel texted me at 11 PM: "I know all the theory. I understand CBT. I can explain DBT skills. But when I'm actually panicking at 2 AM because I can't reach my deployed husband, none of that knowledge helps. I need something I can DO."

She's right. Understanding anxiety doesn't stop panic attacks. Knowing about depression doesn't lift your mood. Reading about coping skills doesn't automatically translate to using them when you're drowning.

Here's the truth about mental health: **You can't think your way out of anxiety. You have to act your way out.**

This chapter is different from the previous ones. We're done with explanations and theory. This is your practical toolkit—specific skills you can use right now, today, when you're overwhelmed, anxious, depressed, angry, or can't sleep.

These aren't "tips" or "suggestions." These are evidence-based techniques that have been tested in research and proven to work. But here's the catch: they only work if you actually practice them.

Reading this chapter won't help you. Practicing these skills will.

Why Skills Practice Actually Matters

Your brain learns through repetition, not through reading. When you're in crisis—when anxiety is spiking, when depression is crushing you, when anger is overwhelming—your thinking brain shuts down. You can't access complex reasoning or remember sophisticated strategies.

What you CAN access are skills you've practiced so many times they've become automatic.

Think about driving a car. When you first learned, you had to consciously think about every step: check mirrors, signal, check blind spot, turn wheel, accelerate. Now? You drive without thinking. Your brain automated the process through repetition.

Mental health skills work the same way. The first time you try a grounding technique during a panic attack, it feels awkward and doesn't work well. But the 20th time? Your body knows what to do. The skill has become automatic.

This is why practicing skills when you're calm is essential. You're building muscle memory so the skills are available when you actually need them.

So here's what I'm asking: Don't just read these skills and think "that makes sense." Actually practice them. Multiple times. Even when you're not in crisis. Especially when you're not in crisis.

Building Your Personal Mental Health Toolkit

Professional tradespeople don't carry every tool ever made. They carry the tools they use most often for their specific work.

Your mental health toolkit should be the same. You don't need to master every skill in this chapter. You need to identify the handful of skills that work for YOUR specific struggles and practice those until they're automatic.

A good personal toolkit includes:

- 2-3 grounding techniques for when you're overwhelmed
- 2-3 anxiety management skills
- 2-3 skills for managing depression
- 1-2 anger management techniques
- 2-3 sleep strategies
- 1-2 resilience-building practices

That's it. Ten to fifteen total skills that you practice regularly. Not 50 skills you've read about once and never use.

As you read through this chapter, mark the skills that resonate with you. Then pick your toolkit skills and commit to practicing them.

Skills for Different Situations: Acute Crisis vs. Ongoing Stress

Not all distress is the same. You need different skills for different situations.

Acute crisis (panic attack, intense rage, immediate overwhelming distress):

- You need skills that work FAST
- Skills that don't require much thinking
- Physical skills that engage your body
- Goal: Reduce intensity from 10/10 to 6/10 so you can function

Ongoing stress (persistent anxiety, chronic depression, sustained anger):

- You need skills that address root causes
- Skills that change thinking patterns or behaviors over time
- Skills you practice regularly, not just in crisis
- Goal: Reduce baseline distress over days and weeks

Military life throws both at you. The phone call that your spouse is injured? Acute crisis. The grinding stress of unemployment and frequent moves? Ongoing stress.

Build your toolkit with skills for both types of situations.

When You're Overwhelmed: Grounding Techniques

Overwhelming distress—whether it's panic, intense fear, or dissociation—requires immediate intervention. Grounding

96

techniques bring you back to the present moment and reduce intensity quickly.

5-4-3-2-1 Grounding Technique

This is the most versatile grounding skill. You can do it anywhere, anytime, without any equipment.

How it works:

- Name **5 things you can see**: Look around. "I see the blue wall, the clock, my coffee mug, the doorway, the chair."

- Name **4 things you can touch**: Actually touch them. "I feel the smooth table, the soft couch fabric, my jeans, my hair."

- Name **3 things you can hear**: Listen. "I hear the air conditioner, traffic outside, my breathing."

- Name **2 things you can smell**: If nothing obvious, smell your shirt, your skin, soap residue on your hands. "I smell laundry detergent, coffee."

- Name **1 thing you can taste**: Actual taste or residual taste. "I taste toothpaste."

Why it works: Panic and overwhelm pull you into your head—into catastrophic thoughts about the future or traumatic memories from the past. Grounding forces your attention to the present moment using your five senses. It interrupts the anxiety spiral.

Practice now: Yes, right now. Do the full 5-4-3-2-1 sequence. Notice how your body feels before and after.

Paired Muscle Relaxation

This technique combines muscle tension with breathing to release physical stress.

How it works:

- Breathe in for 4 counts while tensing a muscle group (fists, shoulders, legs)

- Hold breath and tension for 4 counts

- Breathe out for 6-8 counts while releasing all tension

- Notice the difference between tension and relaxation

- Move through major muscle groups: hands, arms, shoulders, face, chest, stomach, legs, feet

Why it works: When you're overwhelmed, your body holds tension. This technique teaches your body the difference between tension and relaxation, then triggers the relaxation response.

When to use: When you notice physical tension accompanying emotional overwhelm. Particularly good before bed when tension is preventing sleep.

Paced Breathing

Anxiety and panic trigger rapid, shallow breathing, which makes anxiety worse. Paced breathing interrupts this cycle.

Box Breathing (4-4-4-4):

- Breathe in for 4 counts

- Hold for 4 counts

- Breathe out for 4 counts

- Hold empty for 4 counts

- Repeat for 5 minutes

4-7-8 Breathing:

- Breathe in for 4 counts

- Hold for 7 counts

- Breathe out slowly for 8 counts

- Repeat 4-8 times

Why it works: Slow, controlled breathing activates your parasympathetic nervous system (the "rest and digest" system), which counteracts the fight-or-flight response.

Practice tip: Set a timer for 5 minutes daily and practice paced breathing. Build the habit when you're calm so it's available when you're not.

TIPP Skills (For Acute Distress)

When distress is at 9 or 10 out of 10—when you're having a panic attack, when rage is consuming you, when you're dissociating—you need skills that work immediately and powerfully. TIPP skills are designed for exactly these moments.

T - Temperature

Splash your face with cold water or hold ice cubes. The cold activates the dive reflex, which slows your heart rate and calms your nervous system.

How: Fill a bowl with ice water. Hold your breath and dunk your face for 15-30 seconds. Or hold ice cubes in your hands. Or take a cold shower.

I - Intense Exercise

Do intense physical activity for 10-15 minutes: sprint, jump rope, do jumping jacks, run stairs.

Why it works: Intense exercise burns off stress hormones (adrenaline and cortisol) that fuel panic and rage. Your body thinks you've fled the danger or fought the threat, so it can stand down.

P - Paced Breathing

Use the breathing techniques above.

P - Paired Muscle Relaxation

Tense and release muscle groups as described above.

When to use TIPP: When you're at maximum distress. When other skills aren't working. When you need immediate intensity reduction.

Military spouse application: Keep ice packs in your freezer specifically for this. When you get a scary call about your spouse, when you're triggered by secondary trauma, when deployment fear spikes to panic—TIPP skills can bring you down from 10/10 to manageable levels.

When You're Anxious: Managing Worry and Fear

Anxiety is future-focused. Your brain is catastrophizing about what might happen. These skills address anxious thinking patterns and behaviors.

Challenging Anxious Thoughts (CBT)

Anxiety generates thoughts that feel true but aren't necessarily accurate. This technique teaches you to examine evidence.

Step 1: Identify the anxious thought "My husband is going to get killed on this deployment."

Step 2: Rate how much you believe it (0-100%) 85% - feels very true

Step 3: Ask yourself these questions:

- What's the evidence FOR this thought? "Deployments are dangerous. People do die."

- What's the evidence AGAINST this thought? "Most service members return safely. He's well-trained. Statistically, the risk is lower than it feels."

- Am I confusing a feeling with a fact? "I feel terrified, which makes danger feel inevitable. But feelings aren't facts."

- Am I engaging in fortune-telling? "I'm predicting the worst outcome as if it's certain. I don't actually know what will happen."

- What would I tell a friend having this thought? "I'd remind her that fear is understandable but not evidence."

Step 4: Generate a more balanced thought "Deployments involve real risk, and my fear makes sense. But statistically, most service members return safely. I can't control what happens, but I can control how I cope with uncertainty."

Step 5: Re-rate belief in original anxious thought Maybe now it's 40% instead of 85%. That's progress.

Important: The goal isn't to eliminate anxiety completely. The goal is to reduce it from overwhelming to manageable by questioning catastrophic thoughts.

Worry Postponement

When anxiety shows up at inconvenient times (middle of the night, during work, while caring for kids), worry postponement lets you acknowledge the anxiety without being consumed by it.

How it works:

- When anxious thoughts start, say: "I hear you, anxiety. These worries matter. But right now isn't the time to address them. I'm going to think about this during my designated worry time."

- Schedule 15-30 minutes daily as "worry time" (same time each day)

- When worry time arrives, let yourself worry freely for that period

- Keep a worry log if helpful

- When time is up, move on with your day

Why it works: Anxiety thrives on the belief that you MUST address it immediately. Postponement teaches your brain that worry isn't an emergency requiring immediate attention. Paradoxically, when people practice this, they often find they don't need the full worry time—the urgency has decreased.

Mindfulness for Anxiety

Anxiety pulls you into the future. Mindfulness anchors you in the present.

Quick Mindfulness Practice (3 minutes):

- Sit comfortably

- Notice your breath—not changing it, just observing

- When your mind wanders to anxious thoughts (and it will), gently note: "That's an anxious thought"

- Return attention to breath

- Repeat: notice thought, label it, return to breath

Why it works: You're training your brain to observe anxious thoughts without getting hooked by them. The thought "What if something terrible happens?" can just be a thought passing through, not a command to panic.

Behavioral Experiments

Anxiety tells you lies about what will happen. Behavioral experiments test those predictions.

Example: Anxiety says: "If I don't check my phone every 10 minutes during deployment, I'll miss an emergency message and it will be catastrophic."

Experiment: Go 2 hours without checking phone. What actually happens?

Result: Nothing catastrophic. You check after 2 hours, and there's nothing urgent. Or there IS a message, but it waited just fine for 2 hours.

What you learn: Your anxiety was lying about the necessity of constant checking.

How to design experiments:

- Identify what anxiety predicts will happen
- Test the prediction in a controlled way
- Observe actual results
- Compare prediction to reality
- Adjust your behavior based on evidence, not anxiety

When You're Depressed: Activating Your Way Out

Depression says: "Stay in bed. Don't engage. Wait until you feel better." But isolation and inactivity make depression worse. These skills help you act your way out of depression.

Behavioral Activation

This is the most powerful anti-depression skill. The research backing it is solid—behavioral activation works as well as antidepressants for many people with depression.

How it works:

- Schedule activities even when you don't feel like it
- Track your mood before and after activities
- Notice that your mood often improves after engagement, even when you didn't want to do it beforehand
- Use the data to override depression's lies

Types of activities to schedule:

Necessary activities: Things that must get done (shower, grocery shopping, paying bills)

Enjoyable activities: Things you used to enjoy or might enjoy (reading, crafts, cooking, time with friends)

Accomplishment activities: Tasks that create a sense of achievement (organizing a closet, learning something new, completing a project)

Social activities: Any interaction with others (coffee date, phone call, support group)

Physical activities: Movement of any kind (walk, yoga, dancing, gardening)

Create a weekly behavioral activation plan:

Monday:

- Morning: 20-minute walk (mood before: 3/10, after: 5/10)
- Afternoon: Call a friend (mood before: 4/10, after: 6/10)
- Evening: Cook a real meal (mood before: 4/10, after: 5/10)

Track your mood before and after each activity on a 0-10 scale. You'll probably notice a pattern: activities improve mood more often than not, even when depression said they wouldn't.

The behavioral activation rule: Do the activity BEFORE you feel motivated. Motivation follows action, not the other way around.

Opposite Action

Depression urges you to isolate, stay in bed, avoid people, quit activities. Opposite action means doing the opposite of what depression wants.

Depression urge: Stay home from the spouse support group
Opposite action: Go anyway, even though you don't feel like it

Depression urge: Skip the gym because you're too tired **Opposite action:** Go for even 10 minutes

Depression urge: Don't answer texts because you don't have energy for conversation **Opposite action:** Send one brief reply

Why it works: Acting according to depression maintains depression. Acting opposite to depression breaks the cycle.

Important: Start small. If depression says "stay in bed all day," opposite action doesn't mean running a marathon. It means getting out of bed and taking a shower. Build gradually.

Cognitive Restructuring for Depression

Depression generates specific types of distorted thinking. Learning to recognize and challenge these helps lift depressive mood.

Common depression thoughts:

"Nothing ever works out for me." (Overgeneralization)

- Challenge: "That's not true. Some things have worked out. I'm making one situation into all situations."

- More balanced: "This particular situation is hard. Other situations have had different outcomes."

"I'm worthless." (Labeling)

- Challenge: "That's a mean, inaccurate label. I'm a human being with strengths and weaknesses."

- More balanced: "I'm struggling right now, which doesn't determine my worth as a person."

"This will never get better." (Fortune-telling)

- Challenge: "I'm predicting the future based on current feelings. Feelings change."

- More balanced: "Right now, things are hard. I don't know what the future holds. Depression makes me pessimistic, but that doesn't make the pessimism accurate."

Write down your depressive thoughts. Challenge them. Generate alternatives. Depression thrives on unchallenged negative thinking.

Self-Compassion Practices

Depression makes you cruel to yourself. Self-compassion is the antidote.

Self-compassion break (when you're struggling):

- Put your hand on your heart

- Say: "This is a moment of suffering. Suffering is part of life. Many people feel this way. May I be kind to myself. May I give myself the compassion I need."

Sounds cheesy? Try it anyway. Physical touch (hand on heart) combined with kind words activates the care-giving system in your brain, which counteracts depression.

Self-compassion questions:

- "What would I say to a friend feeling this way?"

- "Am I treating myself with the kindness I deserve?"

- "Can I acknowledge my pain without judging myself for it?"

Depression wants you to be harsh with yourself. Self-compassion refuses.

When You're Angry or Frustrated: Managing Intense Emotion

Military life generates legitimate anger. PCS disruptions, spouse unemployment, deployment separations, broken military systems— all anger-inducing. These skills help you manage anger without suppressing it or letting it control you.

STOP Skill

When anger is spiking and you're about to do something you'll regret (yell at your kids, send an angry text, slam doors), use STOP:

S - Stop: Freeze. Don't move. Don't speak.

T - Take a step back: Physically step back if possible. Mentally, step back from the situation.

O - Observe: Notice what's happening. "I'm furious. My heart is racing. I want to yell. I'm having thoughts about how unfair this is."

P - Proceed mindfully: Make a choice about how to respond, rather than reacting impulsively.

Example: Your spouse calls to say the deployment is extended another 3 months. You're furious. You want to scream at him (even though it's not his fault). STOP:

- **Stop:** Don't speak yet

- **Take a step back:** "I need a minute before we talk about this"

- **Observe:** "I'm enraged. I'm having thoughts about quitting this military life. I want to blame him even though this isn't his choice."

- **Proceed mindfully:** "I'm really angry about this news. I need time to process before we discuss it. Can I call you back in 30 minutes?"

STOP creates space between impulse and action. That space is where you regain control.

Opposite Action for Anger

Anger urges you to attack: yell, blame, break things, send mean messages. Opposite action means doing the opposite.

Anger urges: Yell at your kids because you're stressed about deployment **Opposite action:** Take a timeout, calm yourself, then address the situation gently

Anger urges: Send a nasty text to the person who triggered you **Opposite action:** Wait 24 hours, then send a calm, assertive message if still needed

Anger urges: Slam doors, throw things **Opposite action:** Do intense exercise (which burns anger energy without destruction)

Important: Opposite action doesn't mean suppressing anger. It means expressing anger in ways that don't create harm or regret.

Assertive Communication

Anger often masks hurt, fear, or unmet needs. Assertive communication expresses those underlying feelings clearly.

Aggressive communication: "You never help with anything! You're selfish and useless!"

Passive communication: *Says nothing, seethes internally*

Assertive communication: "I'm feeling overwhelmed managing everything alone. I need more help with childcare and household tasks. Can we make a plan for how to share responsibilities?"

Formula for assertive communication:

- "I feel _____ (emotion)"
- "When _____ (specific situation)"
- "I need _____ (request)"

Example: "I feel frustrated when plans change at the last minute because it disrupts everything I've organized. I need as much advance notice as possible about schedule changes."

Assertiveness lets you express anger's underlying message without attacking.

Problem-Solving for Anger Triggers

Sometimes anger signals a problem that needs solving. Use structured problem-solving:

Step 1: Define the problem specifically "I'm angry because military spouse unemployment is affecting our finances"

Step 2: Brainstorm possible solutions (don't judge them yet)

- Remote work opportunities
- Contract/freelance work
- Side income from hobby
- Reduce expenses
- Spouse works extra hours
- Seek financial assistance programs

Step 3: Evaluate each option *List pros and cons of each*

Step 4: Choose solution and make action plan "I'll apply for 5 remote positions this week and research freelance opportunities in my field"

Step 5: Implement and evaluate *After trying, assess: Is this helping? Do I need to try a different solution?*

Problem-solving channels anger into productive action.

When You Can't Sleep: Insomnia Strategies

Sleep problems plague military spouses. Deployment anxiety, rotating schedules, time zone differences, secondary trauma nightmares—all disrupt sleep. These strategies help.

Sleep Hygiene: Military Spouse Edition

Standard sleep hygiene advice doesn't always fit military life. Here's the adapted version:

What you CAN control:

Consistent wake time: Even if bedtime varies (because your spouse calls at weird hours, because kids wake you up), try to wake at the same time daily. This regulates your circadian rhythm.

Bedroom environment: Dark, cool, quiet. Use blackout curtains. White noise machine to cover military housing noise or sudden sounds that trigger hypervigilance.

Pre-bed routine: 30-60 minutes of calming activities before bed. No screens (or use blue light filters if you must check for deployment messages).

Limit caffeine after 2 PM: Caffeine has a 6-hour half-life. That afternoon coffee still affects you at bedtime.

What's harder to control (so give yourself grace):

Regular bedtime: When your spouse calls from deployment at 11 PM, you're taking that call. When kids are sick, sleep gets disrupted. This is reality. Don't beat yourself up.

Worry-free mind: Deployment anxiety doesn't shut off at bedtime. You'll need additional strategies (below).

Managing Deployment-Related Insomnia

Challenge middle-of-night catastrophizing:

When you wake at 3 AM convinced something terrible happened:

Anxious thought: "He hasn't messaged in 36 hours. Something's wrong."

Challenge: "Lack of communication doesn't mean catastrophe. Communication gaps are normal in deployment. I've thought this before and been wrong."

Balanced thought: "I don't know why he hasn't messaged. Most likely explanations are: mission schedule, technology issues, or he's busy. Worrying won't help. I'll check in the morning."

Set a worry appointment: "I acknowledge this concern. I'll think about it tomorrow at 9 AM if it still seems important. Right now, I'm going to sleep."

Cognitive Strategies for Nighttime Rumination

When your brain won't shut off:

Mental categories game: Pick a category (U.S. states, animals, foods) and name items alphabetically. Alabama, Alaska, Arizona... This occupies your thinking mind with something neutral.

Body scan meditation: Focus attention slowly through your body: toes, feet, ankles, calves, knees, thighs, etc. When your mind wanders to worries, gently return to body scan.

Counting backward: Count backward from 300 by 3s. Requires enough attention to prevent rumination but not so much that it wakes you fully.

Get up rule: If you're awake 20+ minutes ruminating, get up. Do something boring (read something dull, fold laundry) until drowsy. Then return to bed. Don't lie in bed strengthening the "bed = anxiety" association.

For Building Resilience: Long-Term Practices

These aren't crisis skills. These are practices you build into your life to increase baseline resilience over time.

Gratitude Practice (Without Toxic Positivity)

Research shows gratitude improves wellbeing. But military spouses hear "be grateful" as a way to dismiss their struggles. That's toxic positivity.

Toxic positivity: "Just be grateful your spouse is alive!"

Authentic gratitude: "Military life is genuinely hard AND I can notice moments of goodness within the difficulty."

How to practice gratitude authentically:

Write three specific things daily:

- One thing that made you smile

- One small pleasure you experienced

- One person you appreciated today

Notice these don't require big positive events. Small moments count: "Good coffee this morning. Sunny weather. Friend texted to check in."

You're not dismissing your struggles. You're training your brain to notice positive experiences that exist alongside hardship.

Meaning-Making

Humans cope better with hardship when they find meaning in it. You can't always choose your circumstances, but you can sometimes choose what they mean.

Questions for meaning-making:

- "What have I learned from military life challenges?"

- "How have I grown through these difficulties?"

- "What values am I living out by handling these struggles?"

- "What matters most to me, and how can I honor that within my circumstances?"

Example: "I didn't choose military spouse unemployment. But managing this has taught me adaptability, resourcefulness, and that my worth isn't tied to a job title. I value personal growth, and I'm growing through this challenge."

Meaning-making doesn't make hardship pleasant. It makes it more bearable.

Post-Traumatic Growth Framework

Not everyone who experiences trauma develops only problems. Many people also experience growth. Research identifies five areas of post-traumatic growth:

1. Personal strength: "I'm stronger than I thought"

2. New possibilities: "This opened doors I wouldn't have seen otherwise"

3. Improved relationships: "I know who my real friends are. I'm closer to the people who matter."

4. Appreciation of life: "I don't take things for granted anymore"

5. Spiritual development: "I've connected with something larger than myself"

Reflection:

- Which growth areas have you experienced?
- How have military life challenges changed you for the better (even alongside the difficulties)?
- What strengths have you discovered in yourself?

Growth and struggle coexist. Acknowledging growth doesn't erase pain, but it adds dimension to your story.

Building Your Support Network Map

Resilience requires support. Map your support system:

Draw circles representing different support types:

Inner circle: People you can call at 2 AM in crisis **Second circle:** Close friends you see/talk to regularly **Third circle:** Good acquaintances, friendly connections **Outer circle:** Professional support (therapist, medical providers) **Virtual layer:** Online connections

Who's in each circle? Are your circles balanced? Do you need to invest in building more support in any area?

Update this map periodically, especially after PCS moves.

Making Skills Practice Sustainable in Chaos

Military life is chaotic. Skills practice must fit into that chaos or it won't happen.

Strategies for sustainable practice:

Anchor practice to existing habits: Practice paced breathing while brushing teeth. Do gratitude journaling while drinking morning coffee.

Start absurdly small: 2 minutes of mindfulness daily beats 30 minutes you never do.

Use reminders: Phone alerts for skills practice. Sticky notes with skill reminders.

Track practice: Use a simple tracker (below). Seeing progress motivates continued practice.

Be flexible: If today's planned skill doesn't fit the situation, use a different one. Practice counts even when it's not perfect.

Batch practice: Dedicate 10 minutes daily to skills practice rather than spreading throughout day.

Skills Don't Replace Therapy: When to Seek Professional Help

These skills help many people significantly. But they're not a substitute for professional treatment when you need it.

Seek professional help when:

- Symptoms are severe (significant depression, panic attacks, PTSD symptoms)
- Symptoms persist despite consistent skills practice

- You're having thoughts of suicide or self-harm

- You're struggling to function in daily life

- Relationship problems are significant

- You need medication evaluation

- You want help from someone with expertise

Skills are like over-the-counter medication—they help with mild to moderate symptoms. Professional therapy is like prescription medication and specialized care—needed for more significant problems.

There's no shame in needing professional help. Military OneSource offers free counseling. TRICARE covers mental health treatment. Use these resources.

Your Personal Crisis Plan

Having a plan for when you're in acute distress helps you access skills when your thinking brain shuts down.

Build your crisis plan:

My warning signs I'm heading toward crisis:

- (Example: "Not sleeping, crying frequently, avoiding people, intrusive thoughts increasing")

My acute crisis skills (in order to try):

1. TIPP skills (ice/cold water)

2. Paced breathing (4-7-8 technique)

3. 5-4-3-2-1 grounding

4. Call support person

My support people and phone numbers:

1. (Friend): 555-1234

2. (Family member): 555-5678

3. Military OneSource: 800-342-9647

4. Crisis Hotline: 988

Professional help if needed:

- My therapist: (name and number)

- Nearest emergency room: (location)

- Suicide & Crisis Lifeline: 988

Keep this plan on your phone and in a physical location you can access in crisis.

Skills Practice Log

Track your skills practice for 2 weeks:

Date	Skill Practiced	Duration	Mood Before (0-10)	Mood After (0-10)	Notes

Use this data. Which skills consistently help? Those become your go-to skills. Which don't help much? Deprioritize those.

"If-Then" Planning for Common Triggers

Plan ahead for predictable triggers:

If I get a scary call about my spouse during deployment, **then** I will use TIPP skills (ice and intense exercise) before checking social media or calling everyone I know.

If I start ruminating about deployment at 2 AM, **then** I will do the mental categories game for 10 minutes before deciding whether to get out of bed.

If I feel anger spiking during an argument, **then** I will use STOP skill and take a 15-minute break before continuing the conversation.

If I notice depression urging me to cancel social plans, **then** I will use opposite action and go anyway.

Write your own if-then plans for your common triggers. This creates automatic action plans that bypass the need for decision-making in difficult moments.

Creating Your Portable Wellness Kit

Build a physical kit you can take during PCS moves:

Digital components:

- Photos of support people
- Relaxing music playlist
- Guided meditation apps
- Crisis numbers in phone
- Skills reminder notes

Physical components:

- Small notebook for journaling
- Fidget items for grounding
- Essential oils for sensory calming
- Photos of happy memories
- Handwritten notes from loved ones
- Comfort items (special mug, soft scarf, etc.)

This kit travels with you, providing comfort and coping tools at every duty station.

What You've Gained

You now have a toolkit of evidence-based skills for managing the full range of military spouse mental health challenges.

When you're overwhelmed: TIPP skills, grounding techniques, paced breathing **When you're anxious:** Cognitive challenging, worry postponement, behavioral experiments **When you're depressed:** Behavioral activation, opposite action, self-compassion **When you're angry:** STOP skill, assertive communication, problem-solving **When you can't sleep:** Sleep hygiene, cognitive strategies, managing deployment anxiety **For building resilience:** Gratitude, meaning-making, post-traumatic growth, support mapping

But here's the truth: Having these skills in your head doesn't help. **Practicing these skills consistently creates real change.**

Start with two or three skills that resonate most. Practice them daily for two weeks. Track your experience. Notice what helps.

Then add another skill. Then another. Build your toolkit gradually until you have reliable go-to strategies for every type of distress you encounter.

The chaos of military life will continue. The deployments, moves, unemployment, isolation—those challenges won't disappear. But your ability to cope with them can transform dramatically.

Small skills, practiced consistently, create significant change over time. Not overnight. But over weeks and months, you'll notice you're handling challenges better. The panic attacks are less frequent. The depression lifts slightly. The anger doesn't control you as much. The sleep improves.

These skills are tools. Use them. Practice them. Let them become automatic. They're yours forever, and they travel with you wherever military life takes you.

Chapter 8: Rooted While Mobile

Maintaining Wellness in Military Life Long-Term

Jessica sat in my office for what she thought might be our last session. She'd been working with me for eight months, and she'd made remarkable progress.

"I feel like a different person," she said. "Eight months ago, I couldn't get out of bed most days. I was having panic attacks multiple times a week. I'd convinced myself I was failing at everything. Now? I'm still dealing with military life challenges, but I'm actually coping. I have skills that work. I have support I can count on. I feel... capable."

She paused. "But I'm terrified. What happens when I stop coming to therapy? What happens at the next PCS? What happens when the next deployment comes? What if I slide backward?"

Jessica was asking the question every person in therapy eventually asks: **How do I maintain wellness after I stop actively working on it?**

This chapter answers that question. You've learned the skills. You've practiced the strategies. You've made progress. Now we need to talk about how to sustain that progress through ongoing military life challenges.

Because here's the reality: Military life doesn't stop throwing challenges at you. You don't reach a point where everything is easy forever. You reach a point where you have tools to handle challenges better—and then you need to keep using those tools.

Progress Review: Look How Far You've Come

Before we talk about maintenance, I want you to acknowledge your progress.

Pull out the assessments you completed in Chapter 1. Look at your scores:

119

- PHQ-9 (depression screening)

- GAD-7 (anxiety screening)

- 8 Dimensions Wellness Inventory

Now complete them again:

PHQ-9 (Depression Screening) - Current

Over the last two weeks, how often have you been bothered by: (0 = Not at all, 1 = Several days, 2 = More than half the days, 3 = Nearly every day)

1. Little interest or pleasure in doing things ___

2. Feeling down, depressed, or hopeless ___

3. Trouble falling/staying asleep or sleeping too much ___

4. Feeling tired or having little energy ___

5. Poor appetite or overeating ___

6. Feeling bad about yourself or that you're a failure ___

7. Trouble concentrating on things ___

8. Moving or speaking slowly, or being fidgety/restless ___

9. Thoughts that you'd be better off dead or of hurting yourself ___

Total now: _____ Total in Chapter 1: _____ Difference: _____

GAD-7 (Anxiety Screening) - Current

Over the last two weeks, how often have you been bothered by: (0 = Not at all, 1 = Several days, 2 = More than half the days, 3 = Nearly every day)

1. Feeling nervous, anxious, or on edge ___

2. Not being able to stop or control worrying ___

3. Worrying too much about different things ___

4. Trouble relaxing ___

5. Being so restless that it's hard to sit still ___

6. Becoming easily annoyed or irritable ___

7. Feeling afraid as if something awful might happen ___

Total now: ___ Total in Chapter 1: ___ Difference: ___

8 Dimensions Wellness Inventory - Current

Rate yourself honestly (1 = struggling significantly, 10 = thriving):

1. Physical wellness ___

2. Emotional wellness ___

3. Social wellness ___

4. Intellectual wellness ___

5. Occupational wellness ___

6. Spiritual wellness ___

7. Environmental wellness ___

8. Financial wellness ___

Total now: ___/80 Total in Chapter 1: ___/80 Difference: ___

Look at those differences. Even small improvements matter. A 2-point decrease in depression or anxiety is meaningful. A 5-point increase in overall wellness is significant.

You did that. Through practicing skills, building support, challenging thoughts, and taking action—you created change.

Celebrating Your Growth (Without Minimizing Ongoing Challenges)

Military spouse culture makes celebration difficult. There's always something harder happening to someone else. There's always another challenge around the corner. Celebrating your growth can feel like tempting fate.

But you need to celebrate anyway.

What does celebration look like?

Naming your growth specifically:

Write down concrete examples:

- "I used STOP skill during an argument instead of yelling"

- "I went to the spouse event even though I felt anxious, and I actually connected with someone"

- "I asked for help when I needed it instead of suffering silently"

- "I stayed in bed only one day this month instead of five"

- "I challenged my catastrophic deployment thoughts instead of spiraling"

Acknowledging your effort:

Change didn't happen automatically. You worked for it. You practiced skills even when they felt awkward. You showed up to therapy even when you didn't feel like it. You kept trying even when progress felt slow.

That effort matters. Acknowledge it: "I worked hard on my mental health, and I'm proud of that effort."

Sharing with safe people:

Tell someone who will celebrate with you. Not to brag, but to let yourself be seen and valued for your growth.

Important: Celebrating growth doesn't mean pretending challenges are over. You can acknowledge both: "I've made significant progress AND military life is still hard. Both are true."

Maintaining Wellness During Ongoing Stressors

Here's the challenge: The stressors that contributed to your depression or anxiety don't stop when you feel better.

Deployments will still happen. PCS moves will continue. Spouse unemployment may persist. Secondary trauma doesn't disappear because you've been to therapy.

So how do you maintain wellness while still facing difficult circumstances?

1. Lower your expectations for "wellness"

Wellness in military life doesn't mean perpetual happiness. It means:

- Managing symptoms so they don't interfere with functioning
- Having bad days without falling into bad months
- Knowing how to cope when challenges spike
- Bouncing back from setbacks more quickly

2. Accept that symptoms fluctuate

You'll have periods of lower symptoms and periods when they spike. That's normal. A spike doesn't mean you've lost all progress—it means you're in a difficult period and need to increase coping efforts.

3. Match your coping intensity to your stress level

During calm periods: Maintenance-level skills practice (10-15 minutes daily)

During moderate stress (PCS move, work stress): Increased skills practice (20-30 minutes daily), maybe extra therapy session

During high stress (deployment, crisis): Intensive coping (multiple skills daily, weekly therapy, increased support)

Think of it like physical fitness. You maintain with regular exercise. When training for a race, you increase intensity. When injured, you modify. Same with mental health.

4. Keep using skills even when you feel good

The biggest mistake people make: stopping skills practice when symptoms improve.

Skills practice when you feel good maintains your improvement. Stopping practice invites relapse.

Continue daily skills practice even during good periods. Think of it as preventive maintenance.

Creating Sustainable Self-Care in a Life That Prioritizes Everyone Else

Military spouse life constantly demands you prioritize others: your service member, your children, your household, your volunteer commitments, your service member's career.

Self-care gets deprioritized. Then you burn out. Then you're no good to anyone.

Sustainable self-care isn't selfish—it's strategic.

What sustainable self-care actually looks like:

Not this: Elaborate self-care routines requiring hours daily that you'll abandon within a week

But this: Small, consistent practices built into your existing routine

Examples of sustainable self-care for military spouses:

5-minute morning practice: Coffee or tea in silence before anyone else wakes. Just 5 minutes of peace.

Phone-free time: One hour daily with phone on silent (unless deployment requires availability). Present with yourself or your family.

Movement: 20-minute walk, yoga video, dance in your kitchen. Not marathon training—just movement.

Social connection: One coffee date or phone call weekly with a friend. Scheduled and protected.

Therapy maintenance: Monthly therapy sessions even when you're "fine" to prevent backsliding.

Hobby time: One hour weekly doing something purely for enjoyment. Reading, crafting, cooking, gaming—whatever brings you pleasure.

Sleep protection: Prioritizing adequate sleep by protecting bedtime routine, even when it's inconvenient.

Boundary-setting: Saying no to commitments that drain you without adding value.

Self-compassion moments: Brief self-compassion breaks throughout the day when you're struggling.

Notice what's missing from this list: expensive spa days, luxury vacations, hours of uninterrupted alone time. Those things are nice when available, but they're not sustainable for most military spouses.

Sustainable self-care fits into military life chaos. It's small, consistent, and non-negotiable.

Warning Signs You're Sliding Backward

You need to know your personal warning signs that symptoms are increasing so you can intervene early.

Common warning signs:

Sleep changes: Sleeping much more or less than usual, nightmares increasing

Appetite changes: Eating much more or less, stopping regular meals

Social withdrawal: Canceling plans, avoiding people, not responding to messages

Irritability: Snapping at people, low frustration tolerance, anger spikes

Loss of interest: Activities you usually enjoy feel pointless

Difficulty concentrating: Can't focus on tasks, mind constantly wandering, making more mistakes

Increased substance use: Drinking more, using substances to cope

Neglecting self-care: Skipping showers, not changing clothes, letting hygiene slip

Stopping skills practice: No longer using coping strategies that helped

Hopelessness: Thoughts like "nothing will ever get better" or "what's the point?"

Physical symptoms: Headaches, stomach issues, tension, fatigue

Create your personalized warning signs list:

Think about previous depressive or anxious episodes. What were the early signs before you were in crisis?

My personal warning signs:

1. _____

2. _____

3. _____

4. _____

5. _____

Share this list with someone close to you. Ask them to gently point out if they notice these signs.

Normalizing Setbacks and Having a Plan

You will have setbacks. This is guaranteed.

A setback doesn't mean failure. It means you're human facing ongoing challenges.

Common setback triggers for military spouses:

- Deployment announcement
- PCS orders
- Job loss or rejection
- Military system frustrations
- Holiday season
- Service member mental health crisis
- Financial emergency
- Relationship conflict
- Isolation at new duty station
- Secondary trauma exposure
- Anniversaries of difficult events

When you have a setback:

Don't catastrophize: "I'm back at square one" is rarely true. You still have skills and knowledge.

Assess objectively: What happened? What triggered the setback? How severe is it?

Return to basics: Pull out your skills toolkit. Start practicing your most effective strategies again.

Increase support: Extra therapy session, reach out to friends, post in support group.

Be compassionate: Talk to yourself like you'd talk to a friend: "You're going through something hard. It makes sense you're struggling. You've gotten through this before. You can handle it."

Use your relapse prevention plan (below).

Adjust expectations: You may need to lower your functioning expectations temporarily. That's okay.

Seek professional help if needed: If the setback is severe or persistent, increase professional support.

Setbacks are part of the process, not evidence of failure.

Relapse Prevention Plan

A relapse prevention plan is your roadmap for handling setbacks.

Build yours now, while you're doing well:

Section 1: My Triggers and Warning Signs

What situations typically trigger symptom increases?

- _____
- _____
- _____

What are my early warning signs?

- _____
- _____
- _____

Section 2: My Protective Factors

What helps me stay well?

- _____
- _____
- _____

What skills work best for me?

- _____
- _____
- _____

Who supports me?

- _____
- _____
- _____

Section 3: Action Plan When Warning Signs Appear

Level 1 (mild symptoms returning):

- Increase daily skills practice to 20-30 minutes
- Reach out to one support person
- Review my coping strategies and choose two to focus on this week

Level 2 (moderate symptoms):

- Schedule therapy appointment
- Use skills multiple times daily
- Reach out to support system actively
- Reduce non-essential commitments

- Revisit my crisis plan

Level 3 (severe symptoms):

- Call therapist for urgent appointment

- Call support people and ask for specific help

- Use crisis resources if needed (988, Military OneSource)

- Inform my spouse (if safe to do so) that I'm struggling and need support

- Consider whether medication evaluation needed

Section 4: Emergency Contacts

Therapist: _____ Support person 1: _____ Support person 2: _____

Crisis line: 988 Military OneSource: 800-342-9647

Keep this plan accessible. Review it every few months. Update as circumstances change.

Building Your Ongoing Support System

Wellness isn't sustained alone. You need ongoing support.

Types of support you need:

Professional support:

- Therapist for maintenance sessions (monthly or as needed)

- Medical provider for medication management if applicable

- Chaplain or spiritual advisor if relevant to you

Peer support:

- 2-3 close friends you can be real with

- Military spouse community connections (online or in-person)

- Support group if helpful

Family support:

- Partner (when available and relationship is healthy)
- Family members who understand and support you
- Parenting support network if you have children

Practical support:

- People who can help during crises (watch kids, bring meals, etc.)
- Professional connections for career support
- Financial advisors if needed

Virtual support:

- Online communities that travel with you during PCS
- Long-distance friendships maintained across moves

Map your current support system. Where are the gaps? What type of support do you need more of?

Building support is ongoing work. After each PCS, you'll need to rebuild local support while maintaining virtual connections. Plan for this.

When to Return to Therapy or Increase Support

You don't only need therapy when you're in crisis. Sometimes returning to therapy proactively prevents crisis.

Consider returning to therapy or increasing therapy frequency when:

- Warning signs are appearing
- Major stressor approaching (deployment, PCS, etc.)
- Skills that usually work aren't helping

- Relationship problems are increasing

- You want to work on something specific (trauma processing, deeper issues)

- You feel yourself sliding toward old patterns

- You just need a check-in and tune-up

Think of therapy like dental care. You don't only go when you have a cavity. You go for regular check-ups to prevent cavities.

Many people benefit from:

- **Intensive phase:** Weekly therapy while in crisis or building initial skills

- **Maintenance phase:** Monthly therapy to sustain progress

- **Check-ins as needed:** Returning when stressors increase

There's no shame in ongoing therapy. Military life is chronically stressful. Ongoing support makes sense.

Advocating for Yourself in Military System

Part of maintaining wellness is advocating for your needs within military systems.

How to advocate effectively:

Know your benefits:

- TRICARE mental health coverage

- Military OneSource free counseling

- Family Readiness programs

- Installation family support services

- Spouse preference for federal employment

- MyCAA scholarship for portable careers

Use your resources:

- Don't wait until crisis to access help
- Connect with Military and Family Life Counselors (MFLC) on installation
- Attend family readiness events that are actually helpful
- Access online support when local resources lacking

Speak up about problems:

- When TRICARE providers are inadequate, request different provider
- When wait times are excessive, escalate to patient advocate
- When spouse employment barriers are unfair, connect with advocacy organizations

Connect with advocacy groups:

- Blue Star Families
- National Military Family Association
- Military spouse employment advocacy groups
- Branch-specific spouse organizations

Vote and contact representatives:

- Military spouse unemployment, license portability, and mental health access are policy issues
- Your voice matters in changing systems

You can't fix broken military systems alone. But you can advocate for yourself and contribute to collective advocacy efforts.

Teaching Resilience to Your Children

Your children watch how you cope with military life challenges. Teaching them resilience helps them AND reinforces your own skills.

How to model and teach resilience:

Name emotions: "I'm feeling frustrated about this PCS move. It's okay to have big feelings about hard things."

Model coping skills: "I'm going to take some deep breaths to calm down. Do you want to do it with me?"

Normalize struggle: "PCS moves are hard for everyone. You're not wrong for being sad about leaving your friends."

Teach problem-solving: "What could we do to make this easier? Let's brainstorm together."

Point out their strengths: "You've moved three times and made new friends each time. You're really adaptable."

Maintain routines: Consistency in bedtime, meals, and family time provides security amid chaos.

Allow their feelings: Don't fix everything or minimize. "You're really sad about daddy deploying. That makes sense."

Age-appropriate involvement: Let them help with PCS decisions or deployment preparation appropriate to their age.

Your wellness directly affects your children's wellness. Taking care of yourself helps them too.

Planning for Transitions: What's Coming Next

Military life involves constant transitions. Planning ahead helps you maintain wellness through them.

Upcoming deployment?

- Review Chapter 2 deployment coping strategies
- Build your support system NOW, before deployment starts

- Increase therapy frequency if needed
- Practice anxiety and distress tolerance skills in advance
- Create communication plan with spouse
- Prep children with age-appropriate information

Upcoming PCS?

- Review Chapter 3 transition strategies
- Start saying goodbyes intentionally
- Build virtual connections before you move
- Research mental health providers at new location
- Pack your portable wellness kit
- Allow yourself to grieve losses
- Create 90-day action plan for new location

Service member separating from military?

- Prepare for identity transition (yours AND theirs)
- Research veteran spouse resources
- Plan for loss of military community
- Connect with veteran spouse networks
- Consider couples therapy to navigate transition together
- Acknowledge this is major change even if it's wanted

Facing multiple stressors simultaneously?

- Lower expectations for functioning
- Increase support significantly
- Use crisis-level coping even though it's not technically "crisis"

- Give yourself permission to just survive rather than thrive temporarily

- Seek professional help proactively

Transitions are predictable stressors. Plan for them rather than being surprised when they're hard.

For Veteran Spouses: Life After Military Transition

Leaving military life is a significant transition with its own challenges:

Identity loss: You were a military spouse for years. Who are you now?

Community loss: You lose built-in military spouse community

Structure loss: Military life, despite frustrations, provided structure

Benefits changes: Transition from TRICARE to other insurance, loss of installation access

Geographic stability: Finally have control over where you live (this is good but requires adjustment)

Partner's transition: Your service member is also transitioning, which affects you

Veteran spouse-specific considerations:

Allow yourself to grieve: Even if you wanted military life to end, you can grieve what you're losing

Build new community: Use geographic stability to invest deeply in local connections

Maintain military spouse friendships: Just because your spouse left military doesn't mean you lose all military spouse friends

Define new identity: Who are you beyond "military spouse"? This is ongoing work.

Seek veteran spouse resources: Blue Star Families includes veteran spouses, some VA programs support caregivers

Consider therapy for transition: This is major life change affecting both partners

The transition out of military life is another challenge to navigate. Use your skills. Seek support. Give yourself time.

Revisiting Our Case Study Characters

Remember Maria, Jennifer, David, Sarah, and Lisa from previous chapters? Here's where they are now—not "fixed," but coping well:

Maria (Army spouse, deployment): Made it through her husband's 12-month deployment using behavioral activation, mindfulness, and support network. Currently preparing for next deployment with less terror because she knows she has tools that work. Depression and anxiety are lower but not gone. She's increased therapy to twice monthly leading up to deployment.

Jennifer (Air Force spouse, PCS): Navigated her fourth PCS move using grief processing and portable toolkit. Still frustrated about career disruption but found meaning through volunteering and online career development. Maintains virtual friendships across duty stations. Practices self-compassion daily.

David (Navy spouse, unemployment/identity): Still underemployed but building freelance engineering consulting work. Redefined success beyond traditional career. Values-aligned activities provide purpose. Depression lifted significantly. Advocates for military spouse employment issues, which channels frustration productively.

Sarah (Guard spouse, isolation): Built hybrid support system of virtual military spouse connections and local civilian friendships. Loneliness decreased from 9/10 to 4/10. Still struggles during husband's training absences but has crisis plan and skills that help. Maintains regular therapy via telehealth.

Lisa (veteran spouse, secondary trauma): Completed trauma-focused therapy for her own secondary traumatic stress. Set boundaries around caregiving for husband with PTSD. Joined veteran spouse support group. Symptoms still present but manageable. Knows warning signs and intervenes early when symptoms increase.

Notice the pattern? None of them are "cured." All still face military life challenges. But they're functioning, coping, and often thriving despite difficulties.

That's realistic recovery. Not perfect, but sustainable.

Your Sustainable Self-Care Menu

Create a menu of self-care options across different time commitments and energy levels. When you need self-care, choose from your menu rather than trying to figure out what to do.

5-minute self-care (when time is severely limited):

- _____

- _____

- _____

15-minute self-care (brief but meaningful):

- _____

- _____

- _____

30-60 minute self-care (moderate time investment):

- _____

- _____

- _____

Low-energy self-care (when depleted):

- _____
- _____
- _____

High-energy self-care (when you have energy to spare):

- _____
- _____
- _____

Social self-care (connection with others):

- _____
- _____
- _____

Solitary self-care (replenishing alone time):

- _____
- _____
- _____

Having options for different circumstances means you can care for yourself even when conditions aren't ideal.

Letter to Yourself: Wisdom for Future Difficult Times

Write a letter to your future self who will inevitably face hard times again. What do you want to remember? What wisdom have you gained?

Dear Future Me,

If you're reading this, you're probably struggling. I'm writing this during a better period so I can remind you of things you might have forgotten.

First, you've been here before. You've felt this bad or worse, and you survived. You have skills now that you didn't have before.

Remember:

[What coping skills work best for you]

[Who your support people are]

[What you've overcome already]

[What gives you hope]

[What you know to be true even when depression/anxiety lies]

You will get through this. Not easily, but you will. Reach out for help. Use your skills. Be compassionate with yourself.

You're stronger than you feel right now.

Love, [Your name]

Keep this letter where you can access it during difficult times.

Resources Guide: Where to Get Help When You Need It

Immediate Crisis:

- 988 Suicide & Crisis Lifeline
- Veterans Crisis Line: 988, then press 1
- Crisis Text Line: Text HOME to 741741
- Military OneSource: 800-342-9647 (24/7)

Mental Health Treatment:

- TRICARE mental health: www.tricare.mil/mentalhealth
- Military OneSource free counseling (12 sessions per issue)
- Military and Family Life Counselors (MFLC) on installation

- Give an Hour (free services from volunteer providers): giveanhour.org

- Vet Centers (for veteran family members): www.va.gov/find-locations

Military Spouse-Specific Support:

- Blue Star Families: bluestarfam.org

- National Military Family Association: militaryfamily.org

- Tragedy Assistance Program for Survivors (TAPS): taps.org

- Military Spouse JD Network (for legal professionals): msjdn.org

Therapy Directories:

- Psychology Today therapist finder: psychologytoday.com

- American Psychological Association: locator.apa.org

- EMDR International Association: emdria.org

- Anxiety and Depression Association of America: adaa.org

Books:

- *The Body Keeps the Score* by Bessel van der Kolk (trauma)

- *Feeling Good* by David Burns (depression and CBT)

- *The Anxiety and Phobia Workbook* by Edmund Bourne

- *Self-Compassion* by Kristin Neff

- *Daring Greatly* by Brené Brown (vulnerability)

Apps:

- Calm or Headspace (mindfulness)

- Sanvello (mood tracking and skills)

- Breathe2Relax (breathing exercises)

- DBT Coach (DBT skills)

- PTSD Coach (trauma symptoms)

Save these resources. Share them with other military spouses who need them.

You Deserve to Thrive, Not Just Survive

We're at the end of this book, but not the end of your journey.

You've learned about the unique mental health challenges military spouses face. You've discovered evidence-based strategies for deployment, PCS moves, career loss, isolation, and secondary trauma. You've built a toolkit of practical skills. You've created plans for maintaining wellness long-term.

But here's what I most want you to remember: **You deserve to thrive, not just survive.**

Military spouse culture glorifies survival. "I made it through another deployment." "I survived another PCS." "I'm hanging in there."

Surviving is good. Surviving matters. But surviving is the minimum standard, not the goal.

You deserve:

- Mental health that's stable, not constantly in crisis

- Relationships that nourish you

- Purpose and meaning in your life

- Joy, not just absence of severe depression

- Peace, not just management of overwhelming anxiety

- Support that actually supports you

- Recognition that your service matters too

Thriving in military life doesn't mean being happy all the time. It means:

- Having skills to cope with challenges effectively
- Maintaining relationships that matter
- Finding purpose despite limitations
- Experiencing joy regularly, not just occasionally
- Managing symptoms so they don't control your life
- Knowing you can handle what comes

You've built the foundation for thriving. Continue building. Keep practicing skills. Maintain support. Advocate for yourself. Seek help when you need it.

Military life will continue throwing challenges at you. Some days will be survival mode. That's okay. But you can have more thriving days than surviving days. You can be rooted even while mobile.

The Skills Are Yours Forever

Here's the beautiful truth: **Every skill you've learned in this book is portable.**

Your therapist at this duty station can't move with you. Your support network will change with every PCS. Your physical environment constantly shifts.

But your skills? Those are yours forever.

The grounding techniques you practiced? Yours. The cognitive restructuring you learned? Yours. The self-compassion you developed? Yours. The behavioral activation that pulled you out of depression? Yours. The boundary-setting that protected your mental health? Yours.

These skills are the most portable things you own. They travel with you to every duty station. They're available during every deployment. They sustain you through every transition.

You built a toolkit that nobody can take from you.

You Can Be Rooted Even While Mobile

The title of this chapter—and this book—promises something that sounds impossible: being rooted while mobile.

How can you be rooted when you move every 2-3 years? When deployments uproot your family? When nothing about military life is stable?

Here's how: **Your roots aren't in the ground. Your roots are inside you.**

Being rooted means:

- Knowing who you are beyond circumstances
- Having values that guide you regardless of location
- Possessing skills that sustain you through transitions
- Maintaining connections that transcend geography
- Finding meaning in your experiences
- Trusting yourself to handle challenges

You can carry that rootedness to every duty station. It travels in your heart, not your moving truck.

You are resilient. Not because military life made you that way (though it certainly tested you), but because you chose to build resilience through deliberate practice and seeking help.

You are rooted. Not in a place, but in yourself.

And you are stronger than you probably give yourself credit for.

Final Words

If you've made it to the end of this book, you've invested significant time and energy in your mental health. That investment matters.

Maybe you read straight through. Maybe you jumped to chapters that addressed your current struggles. Maybe you did every exercise, or maybe you skipped most of them. However you used this book, I hope you found something helpful.

If you take nothing else from these pages, remember this:

You're not broken. You're responding normally to abnormal circumstances. Your struggles are valid. Your mental health matters. Help is available. Recovery is possible. And you deserve better than white-knuckling your way through military life.

Use the skills. Seek support. Be compassionate with yourself. Advocate for change in systems that fail military spouses. Connect with others who understand.

You can do more than survive military life. You can actually live it— with purpose, with connection, with joy alongside the hardships.

You're rooted. You're resilient. And you're exactly where you need to be: taking care of yourself so you can handle whatever comes next.

References

Agllias, K. (2016). Family estrangement: Aberration or common occurrence? *Journal of Family Social Work, 19*(4), 283-294.

Ainsworth, M. D. S., Blehar, M. C., Waters, E., & Wall, S. (1978). *Patterns of attachment: A psychological study of the strange situation*. Lawrence Erlbaum.

Anderson, F. G., Sweezy, M., & Schwartz, R. C. (2017). *Internal family systems skills training manual: Trauma-informed treatment for anxiety, depression, PTSD & substance abuse*. PESI Publishing.

Beck, J. S. (2011). *Cognitive behavior therapy: Basics and beyond* (2nd ed.). Guilford Press.

Blake, L. (2017). Parents and children who are estranged in adulthood: A review and discussion of the literature. *Journal of Family Theory & Review, 9*(4), 521-536.

Boss, P. (1999). *Ambiguous loss: Learning to live with unresolved grief*. Harvard University Press.

Boss, P. (2006). *Loss, trauma, and resilience: Therapeutic work with ambiguous loss*. W. W. Norton & Company.

Bowlby, J. (1988). *A secure base: Parent-child attachment and healthy human development*. Basic Books.

Bradshaw, J. (1988). *Healing the shame that binds you*. Health Communications, Inc.

Bride, B. E., Robinson, M. M., Yegidis, B., & Figley, C. R. (2004). Development and validation of the Secondary Traumatic Stress Scale. *Research on Social Work Practice, 14*(1), 27-35.

Brown, B. (2010). *The gifts of imperfection: Let go of who you think you're supposed to be and embrace who you are*. Hazelden Publishing.

Brown, B. (2012). *Daring greatly: How the courage to be vulnerable transforms the way we live, love, parent, and lead*. Gotham Books.

Burns, D. D. (1980). *Feeling good: The new mood therapy*. William Morrow.

Burns, D. D. (1999). *Feeling good: The new mood therapy*. Avon Books.

Caska, C. M., & Renshaw, K. D. (2011). Perceived burden in spouses of National Guard/Reserve service members deployed during operations Iraqi Freedom and Enduring Freedom. *Journal of Anxiety Disorders, 25*(3), 346-351.

Carr, K., Holman, A., Abetz, J., Kellas, J. K., & Vagnoni, E. (2015). Giving voice to the silence of family estrangement: Comparing reasons of estranged parents and adult children in a nonmatched sample. *Journal of Family Communication, 15*(2), 130-140.

Chapman, A. L. (2006). Dialectical behavior therapy: Current indications and unique elements. *Psychiatry (Edgmont), 3*(9), 62-68.

Coleman, J. (2021). *Rules of estrangement: Why adult children cut ties and how to heal the conflict*. Harmony Books.

Conti, R. P. (2015). Family estrangement: Establishing a prevalence rate. *Journal of Psychology and Behavioral Science, 3*(2), 28-35.

Dekel, R., & Solomon, Z. (2006). Secondary traumatization among wives of Israeli POWs: The role of POWs' distress. *Social Psychiatry and Psychiatric Epidemiology, 41*(1), 27-33.

Department of Veterans Affairs. (2020). Program of Comprehensive Assistance for Family Caregivers. Veterans Health Administration.

Eaton, K. M., Hoge, C. W., Messer, S. C., Whitt, A. A., Cabrera, O. A., McGurk, D., ... & Castro, C. A. (2008). Prevalence of mental health problems, treatment need, and barriers to care among primary care-seeking spouses of military service members involved in Iraq and Afghanistan deployments. *Military Medicine, 173*(11), 1051-1056.

Figley, C. R., & Figley, K. R. (2009). Stemming the tide of trauma systemically: The role of family therapy. *Australian and New Zealand Journal of Family Therapy, 30*(3), 173-183.

Forward, S., & Buck, C. (1989). *Toxic parents: Overcoming their hurtful legacy and reclaiming your life.* Bantam Books.

Gewirtz, A. H., Erbes, C. R., Polusny, M. A., Forgatch, M. S., & DeGarmo, D. S. (2011). Helping military families through the deployment process: Strategies to support parenting. *Professional Psychology: Research and Practice, 42*(1), 56-62.

Gewirtz, A. H., Polusny, M. A., DeGarmo, D. S., Khaylis, A., & Erbes, C. R. (2010). Posttraumatic stress symptoms among National Guard soldiers deployed to Iraq: Associations with parenting behaviors and couple adjustment. *Journal of Consulting and Clinical Psychology, 78*(5), 599-610.

Gibson, L. C. (2015). *Adult children of emotionally immature parents: How to heal from distant, rejecting, or self-involved parents.* New Harbinger Publications.

Harris, R. (2009). *ACT made simple: An easy-to-read primer on acceptance and commitment therapy.* New Harbinger Publications.

Hayes, S. C., & Smith, S. (2005). *Get out of your mind and into your life: The new acceptance and commitment therapy.* New Harbinger Publications.

Hayes, S. C., Strosahl, K. D., & Wilson, K. G. (2011). *Acceptance and commitment therapy: The process and practice of mindful change* (2nd ed.). Guilford Press.

Institute of Medicine. (2013). *Returning home from Iraq and Afghanistan: Assessment of readjustment needs of veterans, service members, and their families.* National Academies Press.

Jacobson, N. S., Martell, C. R., & Dimidjian, S. (2001). Behavioral activation treatment for depression: Returning to contextual roots. *Clinical Psychology: Science and Practice, 8*(3), 255-270.

Kabat-Zinn, J. (2013). *Full catastrophe living: Using the wisdom of your body and mind to face stress, pain, and illness* (Revised ed.). Bantam Books.

Kellerman, N. P. F. (2013). Epigenetic transmission of Holocaust trauma: Can nightmares be inherited? *Israel Journal of Psychiatry and Related Sciences, 50*(1), 33-39.

Knobloch, L. K., & Theiss, J. A. (2012). Experiences of US military couples during the post-deployment transition: Applying the relational turbulence model. *Journal of Social and Personal Relationships, 29*(4), 423-450.

Lambert, J. E., Engh, R., Hasbun, A., & Holzer, J. (2012). Impact of posttraumatic stress disorder on the relationship quality and psychological distress of intimate partners: A meta-analytic review. *Journal of Family Psychology, 26*(5), 729-737.

Lebow, J. L., Chambers, A. L., Christensen, A., & Johnson, S. M. (2012). Research on the treatment of couple distress. *Journal of Marital and Family Therapy, 38*(1), 145-168.

Lester, P., Aralis, H., Sinclair, M., Kiff, C., Lee, K. H., Mustillo, S., & Wadsworth, S. M. (2016). The impact of deployment on parental, family and child adjustment in military families. *Child Psychiatry & Human Development, 47*(6), 938-949.

Lester, P., Peterson, K., Reeves, J., Knauss, L., Glover, D., Mogil, C., ... & Beardslee, W. (2010). The long war and parental combat deployment: Effects on military children and at-home spouses. *Journal of the American Academy of Child & Adolescent Psychiatry, 49*(4), 310-320.

Levine, A., & Heller, R. (2010). *Attached: The new science of adult attachment and how it can help you find—and keep—love.* TarcherPerigee.

Linehan, M. M. (2014). *DBT skills training handouts and worksheets* (2nd ed.). Guilford Press.

Linehan, M. M. (2014). *DBT skills training manual* (2nd ed.). Guilford Press.

Manguno-Mire, G., Sautter, F., Lyons, J., Myers, L., Perry, D., Sherman, M., ... & Sullivan, G. (2007). Psychological distress and burden among female partners of combat veterans with PTSD. *The Journal of Nervous and Mental Disease, 195*(2), 144-151.

Mansfield, A. J., Kaufman, J. S., Marshall, S. W., Gaynes, B. N., Morrissey, J. P., & Engel, C. C. (2010). Deployment and the use of mental health services among US Army wives. *New England Journal of Medicine, 362*(2), 101-109.

Martell, C. R., Dimidjian, S., & Herman-Dunn, R. (2010). *Behavioral activation for depression: A clinician's guide.* Guilford Press.

McBride, K. (2008). *Will I ever be good enough? Healing the daughters of narcissistic mothers.* Free Press.

McKay, M., Wood, J. C., & Brantley, J. (2007). *The dialectical behavior therapy skills workbook: Practical DBT exercises for learning mindfulness, interpersonal effectiveness, emotion regulation, and distress tolerance.* New Harbinger Publications.

Meadows, S. O., Miller, L. L., & Robson, S. (2015). *Airman and family resilience: Lessons from the scientific literature.* RAND Corporation.

Mikulincer, M., & Shaver, P. R. (2007). *Attachment in adulthood: Structure, dynamics, and change.* Guilford Press.

Mmari, K., Roche, K. M., Sudhinaraset, M., & Blum, R. (2009). When a parent goes off to war: Exploring the issues faced by adolescents and their families. *Youth & Society, 40*(4), 455-475.

Monson, C. M., Fredman, S. J., & Dekel, R. (2010). Posttraumatic stress disorder in an interpersonal context. In J. G. Beck (Ed.), *Interpersonal processes in the anxiety disorders: Implications for understanding psychopathology and treatment* (pp. 179-208). American Psychological Association.

Neff, K. D. (2011). *Self-compassion: The proven power of being kind to yourself.* William Morrow.

Orsillo, S. M., & Roemer, L. (2011). *The mindful way through anxiety: Break free from chronic worry and reclaim your life.* Guilford Press.

Porges, S. W. (2011). *The polyvagal theory: Neurophysiological foundations of emotions, attachment, communication, and self-regulation.* W. W. Norton & Company.

Rathus, J. H., & Miller, A. L. (2014). *DBT skills manual for adolescents.* Guilford Press.

Renshaw, K. D., Rodrigues, C. S., & Jones, D. H. (2008). Psychological symptoms and marital satisfaction in spouses of Operation Iraqi Freedom veterans: Relationships with spouses' perceptions of veterans' experiences and symptoms. *Journal of Family Psychology, 22*(4), 586-594.

Resick, P. A., Monson, C. M., & Chard, K. M. (2016). *Cognitive processing therapy for PTSD: A comprehensive manual.* Guilford Press.

Sayers, S. L., Farrow, V. A., Ross, J., & Oslin, D. W. (2009). Family problems among recently returned military veterans referred for a mental health evaluation. *Journal of Clinical Psychiatry, 70*(2), 163-170.

Scharp, K. M. (2020). "You're not welcome here": A grounded theory of family distancing. *Communication Research, 47*(4), 451-471.

Scharp, K. M., & Thomas, L. J. (2016). Family "bonds": Making meaning of parent-child relationships in estrangement narratives. *Journal of Family Communication, 16*(1), 32-50.

Schwartz, R. C. (2001). *Introduction to the internal family systems model*. Trailheads Publications.

Schwartz, R. C. (2021). *No bad parts: Healing trauma and restoring wholeness with the internal family systems model*. Sounds True.

Schwartz, R. C., & Sweezy, M. (2020). *Internal family systems therapy* (2nd ed.). Guilford Press.

Shapiro, F. (2018). *Eye movement desensitization and reprocessing (EMDR) therapy: Basic principles, protocols, and procedures* (3rd ed.). Guilford Press.

Stoddard, J. A., & Afari, N. (2014). *The big book of ACT metaphors: A practitioner's guide to experiential exercises and metaphors in acceptance and commitment therapy*. New Harbinger Publications.

Tedeschi, R. G., & Calhoun, L. G. (2004). Posttraumatic growth: Conceptual foundations and empirical evidence. *Psychological Inquiry, 15*(1), 1-18.

van der Kolk, B. (2014). *The body keeps the score: Brain, mind, and body in the healing of trauma*. Viking.

Verdeli, H., Baily, C., Vousoura, E., Belser, A., Singla, D., & Manos, G. (2011). The case for treating depression in military spouses. *Journal of Family Psychology, 25*(4), 488-496.

Walker, P. (2013). *Complex PTSD: From surviving to thriving*. CreateSpace Independent Publishing Platform.

Webb, J. (2012). *Running on empty: Overcome your childhood emotional neglect*. Morgan James Publishing.

Yehuda, R., & Lehrner, A. (2018). Intergenerational transmission of trauma effects: Putative role of epigenetic mechanisms. *World Psychiatry, 17*(3), 243-257.

Young, J. E., Klosko, J. S., & Weishaar, M. E. (2003). *Schema therapy: A practitioner's guide*. Guilford Press.

www.ingramcontent.com/pod-product-compliance
Lightning Source LLC
Chambersburg PA
CBHW070758290326
41931CB00011BA/2057